THE
HEALTHY
BALANCE

THE
HEALTHY
BALANCE

Cynthia Culp Allen

&

Charity Allen Winters

SPIRE

© 2004 by Cynthia Culp Allen and Charity Allen Winters

Published by Fleming H. Revell
a division of Baker Publishing Group
P.O. Box 6287, Grand Rapids, MI 49516-6287
www.revellbooks.com

Spire edition published 2006
ISBN 10: 0-8007-8739-0
ISBN 978-0-8007-8739-4

Previously published under the title *The Healthy Balance for Body and Soul*

Printed in the United States of America

Unless otherwise indicated, Scripture is taken from the New American Standard Bible®, Copyright © 1960, 1962, 1963, 1968, 1971, 1972, 1973, 1975, 1977, 1995 by The Lockman Foundation. Used by permission.

Scripture marked KJV is taken from the King James Version of the Bible.

Scripture marked NIV is taken from the HOLY BIBLE, NEW INTERNATIONAL VERSION®. NIV®. Copyright © 1973, 1978, 1984 by International Bible Society. Used by permission of Zondervan. All rights reserved.

Scripture marked NKJV is taken from the New King James Version. Copyright © 1982 by Thomas Nelson, Inc. Used by permission. All rights reserved.

Scripture marked NLT is taken from the *Holy Bible*, New Living Translation, copyright © 1996. Used by permission of Tyndale House Publishers, Inc., Wheaton, Illinois 60189. All rights reserved.

Scripture marked TLB is taken from *The Living Bible*, copyright © 1971. Used by permission of Tyndale House Publishers, Inc., Wheaton, Illinois 60189. All rights reserved.

Contents

Acknowledgments 7

1. Health: A Pearl of Great Price 11
2. My Personal Journey to Wellness: Cynthia's Story 29
3. Healthy Balance Foods for Body and Soul 45
4. Lean for Life: The *Healthy Balance* Way 73
5. Recipes for a Healthy Balance 115
6. "I Told You I Was Sick!" 143
7. Feel-Good Fitness for the Total You 179
8. Geared Up for Fitness 211
9. R and R for Life Balance 229
10. The *Healthy Balance* for Life 253

Notes 261
Resources 265

We dedicate this health and fitness book to all the true healers out there—those doctors and nurses and caretakers who
not only have the gift to heal but the heart to heal, and to
all those seekers who, like the leper in Scripture, long to be
healed in body and soul, and to the Great Physician, who
always desires to make them whole.

> Suddenly, a man with leprosy approached Jesus. He knelt
> before Him, worshiping. "Lord," the man said, "if you want
> to, you can make me well again." Jesus touched him. "I want
> to," he said. "Be healed!"

Matthew 8:2-3 NLT

Acknowledgments

From Cynthia: This book, our LifeBalance series, and my ministry are a dream come true for me. For many years, I've had a burning desire to help fellow sufferers by offering them the Truth for body and soul. Little did I realize how long and difficult the process would be. I needed a lot of help along the way and I have many people to thank . . . My mother, mother-in-law, and grandmothers Ray, Garnie, and Jennie (all three now receiving their rewards in heaven) for always coming alongside to help me when I was sick. My dad, who always felt sorry for me but didn't know what to do to help—that's okay, Dad, sometimes all we really want is a little sympathy. My husband for not running off when he finally realized "for better, for worse, in sickness and health" weren't just words mumbled thoughtlessly at the altar. My kids who learned to serve when their mother couldn't serve them—and made me laugh (always good for the immune system!) when there really wasn't anything to laugh about. The churches who became the loving hands of God when I needed them. Drs. Malan, Mulders, and Crook, who reached out of the box to help me. Several friends who joined with me to fight their personal battles against disease—Eileen, Rita, Lori, Phyllis, sisters Sandra and Jill, Pam, Jenny, Sharon, Aunt Sharon, and Aunt Martha. My editorial team at Revell for truly wanting to help their readers in body and soul. Thanks to all those who prayed for me when I so desperately needed prayer. And to Jesus Christ, who has worked more mighty miracles in my life than I deserve, but I'm so grateful that he did—all glory, praise, and honor go to him!

From Charity: With this book, I would like to acknowledge several people in my life who have contributed greatly to the strong, healthy woman I have become in body and soul . . . My dad, Charles Allen, who passed on to me physical health, stamina, and great genes, and who has also passed on to me fortitude of the mind and the life value of self-discipline. My mom, Cynthia Allen, my own personal natural health doctor who has taught me everything she knows about health in this life and about faith for the next. My husband, Kelvin Winters, thank you for continually providing motivation and inspiration to become the best me I can be, but most of all for loving me just as I am. My father-in-law, Reverend Robert Winters, a faithful servant in the body of Christ for over thirty-five years, thank you for the model of devotion to Christ you have been to so many over the years and for the man of faith you continue to be now, in your own courageous battle with illness. Thank you for being a spiritual advisor to us in the writing of this book. We honor you and are greatly blessed by your life! My mother-in-law, MaryBeth Winters, for her inspiring, joyful heart in the midst of great struggle and her unwavering commitment to "stand by her man"! My grandparents, Richard and Geneva Culp and Chuck and Paula Allen, for their support and prayers over the years and for influencing our families to stick together every time "the going gets tough." Our friends and business associates at Revell, Alive Communications, and Planned Television Arts, thank you for your commitment to help us help others. And to my Lord and Savior, Jesus Christ who has been so faithful we want to shout it from the roof tops! I guess this book is our chance!

I

Health

A Pearl of Great Price

How important is health? What amount of money would you be willing to pay to buy health if you could? Would it be worth a million dollars to you? It's a relative question, isn't it? If you are reasonably healthy, you may want to spend your money on something else. If you only suffer with a complaint or two, perhaps you're tired once in a while but overall you're doing fairly well, you might not be willing to shell out as much as someone else. What is wellness worth? Ask patients in hospital cancer wards that same question. Most would agree that they would pay any amount of money to regain their health. Ask the parents of a terminally ill child. A million dollars is a small ransom to pay the disease that has taken their son or daughter hostage.

Health is a priceless possession, more important than the houses, cars, furniture, jewels, and other assets our culture so highly values. Strength and stamina—gifts most of us receive at birth—can be maintained or lost during a lifetime, depending on the receiver's stewardship. The Bible emphasizes good stewardship of the gifts God has given us. In *The Beautiful Balance,* the first book in our LifeBalance series, we featured the maintenance of our physical resources from head to toe, inside and out—our faces, hair, skin, hands, feet, fragrance, and the enhancements we use like cosmetics, wardrobe, and accessories. By applying our advice in that book, you can shine like a beautiful jewel! The same stewardship should be given to all of our assets: brains, talents, health, time, work and ministry, family, home, friends, finances, and relationship with God.

> **The first wealth is health.**
>
> Ralph Waldo Emerson

Adam and Eve were the designated stewards over the Garden of Eden. The *Random House Webster's Dictionary* describes a steward as "a person who manages another's property or finances." The hot property, Eden, belonged to God. Genesis 2:8 says,

> The LORD God planted a garden toward the east, in Eden.

When you're looking in the Yellow Pages for an expert to landscape your new luxury home, you want only the best, right? The Garden's design was created by the world's greatest Landscaper. Think of the most gorgeous scenery you've ever glimpsed (personally or in pictures). Hawaii? No match for this lush paradise. Cancun? A desert in comparison. Fiji? Okay, it could come close, but it still doesn't measure up anymore (thanks to the fall, remember?). Perfect in every way, this tropical nirvana called Eden boasted four sparkling rivers and every species of plant life known to man.

> Out of the ground the LORD God caused to grow every tree that is pleasing to the sight and good for food; the tree

of life also in the midst of the garden, and the tree of the knowledge of good and evil.

Genesis 2:9

Clusters of precious gems were tucked here and there, along with abundant bright flowers. The whole place literally glittered with the colors of the rainbow! Sounds like heaven, doesn't it?

Then the LORD God took the man and put him into the garden of Eden to cultivate and keep it.

Genesis 2:15

After the honeymoon, it was Adam and Eve's job to oversee the development of this incomparable creation. What an awesome privilege and responsibility! On a scale from one to ten, what kind of stewards were they? Minus five! The pair forfeited God's assets to his worst Enemy. By not heeding the Owner's Manual (and doing the exact opposite of God's instruction), the Garden's managers handed the property deed over to Satan. Since then, God's creation—from horticulture to agriculture to human culture—has been on a downward spiral. In the same way, the perfect health and maintenance plan presented in the beginning for our bodies deteriorated, leaving so many of us in the sorry state we're in. But all is not lost. Back in the beginning, God also promised a redeemer. This one, unique Person bought back the deed to Creation with the ultimate ransom: his own blood.

We can know wholeness in body and soul when we commit our lives to Christ's leadership. In *The Healthy Balance,* we'll suggest ways to cultivate a gratifying relationship with the Lord Jesus. Weston A. Price, D.D.S., author of the classic volume *Nutrition and Physical Degeneration,* once said,

"Life in all its fullness is Mother Nature obeyed."[1] As Christians, we know that it's important to obey our Father and Creator. He gives life and breath and holds all of creation in his hands. He designed a strategy for total wellness, and in the following pages, we'll share with you everything we've discovered about his proven health and fitness program. Gone are the leisurely days of the garden, trimming a petunia here, naming an animal there, stopping to smell the roses. Our hectic lives are filled with noise and crowds, confusion, and too much busyness. We'll take a look at how you can gain and maintain physical and psychological health in today's crazy world.

How Important Is Health?

Sometimes we don't realize something's value until we've lost it. (We're sure Adam and Eve experienced this shocker!) A friend we'll call Mary was this way. She possessed a remarkable immune system, one that was faithful to protect her in spite of her assaults on it. A frightening diet of coffee, doughnuts, microwaved goodies, and fast food combined with a sedentary job to pile on the pounds (in spite of the smoking she wouldn't stop because it "kept the weight off"). But she never got sick. Friends and family begged Mary to change her lifestyle. At the time, it didn't matter to her. Today it does, however. She now has cancer. Mary is facing death, and she's urgently searching the Internet for somewhere, anywhere, to find healing.

If good health were a place called Wellbeing, would you be willing to travel there if it were a thousand miles away? Five thousand? Ten thousand? Mary would, because when you lose something important, you desperately want it back.

It becomes the pearl of great price to you. If you are in Mary's shoes, wanting to recapture your vigor, remember the Chinese proverb, "A journey of a thousand miles begins with a single step." Vibrant health may seem out of reach for you now. You believe you are too far gone. But we know you're not. People at death's door have regained their health and even gone to levels they hadn't previously experienced. I (Cynthia) know this from experience. When I lost my health, I had to study extensively to learn how to rebuild my body through nutrition and lifestyle changes. When I began my restorative exercise regimen, I could literally only walk a few steps before I was forced to stop and rest. I have traveled great lengths to regain my health. And I'm still on that journey.

In *The Healthy Balance*, you'll benefit from my experience of losing and recovering my health (in chapter 2). The *Healthy Balance* program presented in this book developed out of years of researching medical journals and health books, brainstorming with physicians and nutritionists, attending medical conferences, consulting with experts, and experimenting on myself and other patients. The *Healthy Balance* plan healed me of an autoimmune disease, cured me of a chronic candida infection, strengthened my immune system, built up my body, and helped me lose extra weight. If you have undiagnosed symptoms and other problems that are plaguing you, this could be your answer. It's a balanced nutrition and exercise plan that also encourages you to find rest for your body and soul. (Take this book to your doctor for his or her approval of the plan before you embark on your adventure in healing.)

We recommend beginning a "New You" notebook to record your journey toward health and wholeness. This notebook will hold your goals and dreams, some important statistics about yourself, the information that will help you reach your objectives, and anything creative that you want to add for motivation. Instructions on making (or ordering) and using this helpful tool are in chapter 8.

True Confessions from Charity

Those who enjoy good health and want to protect it will be encouraged by my story (Charity) of health maintenance and the rewards that result from living the *Healthy Balance* lifestyle.

Remember the television ad in which a gorgeous model stated matter-of-factly, "Don't hate me because I'm beautiful"? She just couldn't help it that she was near perfection. I instantly hated her. How about you? Well, don't hate me because I'm healthy. I really can't help myself. I'm simply the positive by-product of a sick mother who learned how to raise healthy children. And boy, am I ever grateful! Did you have a mother who taught you the principles of living right physically and spiritually? Then you, like me, have much to be grateful for. If that isn't the case for you, we'll share these truths with you in our LifeBalance series. It's never too late to begin your journey toward health for body and soul.

> Prevention is so much better than healing because it saves the labor of being sick.
>
> Thomas Adams,
> 17th-century physician

Are you consistently healthy? Known for your endless energy? Is your idea of being sick catching a cold or flu bug once a year? Are you interested in maintaining your good state of health and high energy level, or perhaps even taking yourself to a higher level? Then you'll identify with me.

> And, I might add, it saves the time! I have wasted years in bed being sick—it's a joy to have the strength to serve God today!
>
> Cynthia Allen

Growing up, it was obvious to me that my parents were two very different people. This was no exception when it came to their health. My dad has always had what our family calls an "iron immune system." The rest of the family could be as sick as dogs, lying in bed moaning and groaning in misery. Meanwhile, Dad would march down the hall, a vision of energy and health, announcing to us everything he planned to get done that day. If sickness was ever going around, Dad was always the last to get it, if he got it at all. I think I could count on one hand the times he actually "caught" something. My dad has been a constant source of strength to me. His physical fortitude has always lined up consistently with his mental and emotional vigor.

My mom, Cynthia, on the other hand, has struggled with ongoing sickness since her teens. Battles with a chronic autoimmune disease often left her bedridden for months (detailed in chapter 2). Frail and vulnerable, Mom was usually the first to catch the "bug" and the last to get rid of it. I recognized that in looks and personality I was a combination of my two parents. Even at a young age, I found myself wondering which parent I would be more like healthwise.

My mother, also concerned, watched me carefully in an attempt to recognize early signs of inherited poor health. Meanwhile, she taught me the importance of staying active, eating healthy, and taking my vitamins religiously. As I grew strong and energetic into my teen years, it became evident that by God's grace and Mom's tutelage, I had been blessed with good health. Not perfect health, mind you. I once had a serious battle with pneumonia that collapsed my lung one summer. Then there was my senior year in high school when I caught an embarrassing case of the chicken pox! Still, my good health seemed consistent. Unlike my mother (bless her heart!), sickness was a rarity for me, not a common occurrence. Thankfully, as my mother developed the *Healthy Balance* lifestyle and committed herself to it, she too has been blessed with amazing health.

Just because I was healthy doesn't mean I was thin and fit, however. In fact, my struggle was not with illness, but with my weight. For several years in my late childhood, I was chubby, and yes, homely for a stage. Echoes of nicknames still ring in my ears from time to time, keeping me forever humble. "Chipmunk Cheeks" and "Bubble Butt" were the kids' favorites. When I was eleven, I dropped out of my beloved gymnastics team after hearing that last name a few too many times.

Energetic as a child, I wanted to be involved in activities and sports. But I couldn't seem to find the right fit for me. I never seemed to stick with anything! This furthered my bad feelings about myself until my Grandma Neva announced one day that my uncle (who was three years older than me) had just joined the town's swim team. She mentioned how much he loved it, and my sad eyes lit up. Maybe swimming would be the activity for me! I loved the water and I loved to swim. I joined that day. I remained on the swim team for eight years. After several weeks of daily swim practice, I had trimmed down my chubby face and bubble butt. In their place were toned muscles. Hooray, I was no longer called "Chipmunk Cheeks"! Finding the right exercise for me was all it took to jump-start my metabolism and teach me to enjoy staying active.

Train up a child in the way he should go,
Even when he is old he will not depart from it.

Proverbs 22:6

This verse in Proverbs has been so true in my life. Growing up, I was taught that there is a healthy way to live physically, emotionally, and spiritually. We ate well, stayed active, and lived a balanced life. Mom taught us God's Word every day and insisted that we live by it. In college, I noticed that my diet and lifestyle were healthier than many of my friends. Now in my late twenties, I still eat nutritiously and cook that way for my new husband. The Lord and his Word are at the center of our marriage. Living five hundred miles away from my family, I'm no longer under Mom's watchful eye. I live this way for me now, because it's the right way. Besides, I've experienced the rewards of a healthy, balanced life. Who wouldn't want to pursue a blessing?

I wrote this journal entry after a rare bout with the flu several years ago:

For over two weeks now I have been sick and bedridden. I have spent hours upon hours, and days upon days staring at the walls. But all of that time I've spent thinking and praying about my life. Oh, how much I have taken for granted, like my health and energy for instance. There is no limit to the things that could be accomplished through my life for God if I would only pair my energy with my strong will combined with my passionate heart. I could do so much more than I have done. It's amazing how the whole world changes when you're thankful . . . the sun is brighter, the air feels

*fresher on your skin, loved ones grow more precious,
sights and smells you've never noticed suddenly catch
your attention. Music ignites your soul and God is
everywhere . . . because now, you are truly alive and
life comes from him. Lord, I will praise you for this gift
of life as long as I have breath to live!*

Chronic Illness in the Body

Unfortunately, good health like this is not the norm.
As we have traveled around the United States speaking to
churches and Christian conferences and camps, we've noticed that there is a record amount of illness in the body of
Christ. People come to us with their distressing symptoms,
many of them practically disabled. Many are still undiagnosed after years of medical care. In most cases, when we ask
about their lifestyles, the reasons for their condition become
obvious. You have to put the correct fuel in the vehicle to
get it to go. I (Cynthia) found this out the hard way once
when I accidentally put diesel in the family car instead of
gasoline. I didn't go anywhere! My unhappy husband had
to come rescue me at the gas station. People are filling up
their tanks with the wrong fuel. They then wonder why the
marvelous machinery called the human body isn't working
right. The church is limping along, unable to serve Christ as
effectively as it could, because so many of us are physically
feeble. Jesus told his followers, "Go into all the world and
preach the gospel to every nation." But today's church has
no get up and go, period. Illness plagues Christ's body.

The church is also sick in soul. Sin-sick, that is. As we
have visited church after church, the stories we have heard

of backslidden lives are grievous. [We must start seeing our spiritual condition through Jesus' eyes if we are to heal his body, the Church.]

Back to Your Body

The apostle Paul made it so clear that our bodies are the temples of the Holy Spirit. In biblical times, there were strict requirements for the building, decorating, and maintaining of the temple. That was the place for God to meet with his family. It was to be kept in tip-top shape. Imagine going to worship each week in a building with mud on the floor, torn-down walls, a roof that leaked, a foul smell, and pigs running in and out. Out of respect for the Lord and his worthiness, and out of gratitude for all he had given, it would behoove the worshipers to first clean up the place.

The Jews polished up the temple so brightly that it was a true reflection of the One whom they worshiped. Physically speaking, it's hard to shine as God's temple when you're feeling shoddy! In some of our lives, we need to do major renovations in body and soul before we do any polishing. That's where this book can help. (If you already enjoy good health, grab *The Beautiful Balance,* the first book in the LifeBalance series. You're ready to do some decorating!)

Scripture gives us examples of saints who maintained their vitality and fitness. Jesus seemed the picture of health as he fulfilled his calling within a three-year time period. In fact, our Lord was the perfect example of a healthy balance. Luke 2:52 says that he grew in "wisdom and stature, and in favor with God and men." Basically, he grew in body and soul. You're not balanced if you grow in one area without the other.

Other examples include Peter and Paul. The disciple Peter clearly lived by the Law's dietary guidelines, so much so that it took a vision for him to see God's nutritious additions. The apostle Paul spoke of the earthly value of physical exercise and disciplined his body for humility and his soul for godliness.

The B.C. *Healthy Balance* Plan

As women seeking health and balance, we have a prototype in Proverbs 31. This virtuous woman is a symbol of perfect health, a condition used for her family's good and God's glory. Proverbia, as we'll call her, is the Martha Stewart of her day. Mercy, that woman had energy! "She never sits still!" verse 27 reads (in the authors' personal translation). From before dawn to long after dusk her day is packed full of activity. She shops far and wide to find the best bargains, weaves and crochets, whips up gourmet meals, buys a field with her own money and plants it, sews clothes for herself, her family, and a few others, develops two businesses, teaches everyone who will listen, runs a household, and volunteers for charity. She's the woman we love to hate!

Where does Ms. Pep get her vim and vigor? Most importantly, she has the fear of the Lord, according to verse 30. The lady knows to put God first because he is the awesome Creator. Proverbia has her priorities straight. She's a balanced gal. In *The Healthy Balance,* we're going to share the blessings of placing Jesus Christ in the center of your life. When you do that, everything else falls into place. When you love, honor, obey, and serve him, you are perfectly balanced in soul. But we are also going to tell you how to be balanced in body. Two lines in verse 17 give away spunky

Proverbia's secret: "She girds herself [literally "her loins"] with strength and makes her arms strong." The virtuous woman works out! The loin area is the middle of the body—you know, the area that "goes to pot" after several children or too many hot fudge sundaes. More than any other area of our bodies, our loins reveal when we are overfed and underexercised. Proverbia strengthens this pelvic area (her God-given natural girdle) with spot-toning exercises. And the other area she works on is her arms. Those of us over forty know this area all too well.

Our judgment of others may be coming back to haunt us. Jesus said, "Do not judge so that you will not be judged . . . by your standard of measure, it will be measured to you" (Luke 6:37–38). It's a basic universal principle: What goes around, comes around. Remember how in junior high we used to laugh at our over-forty female teachers when they wrote on the blackboard? Jiggle, jiggle, jiggle went the loose skin under their arms. Tee-hee—so funny! That will never happen to us. Yeah, right. Now my kids call me (Cynthia) "Chicken Arms"!

Proverbia avoids this vicious name-calling by strengthening her arms. Smart lady. Labels often stick for life. No matter how much I work on my triceps, I'm still "Chicken Arms" to some. In these pages, we'll share exercises to keep your body firm and jiggle-free.

Proverbia's active lifestyle is unprecedented (I mean, who do you know that buys a field and plants a vineyard herself?). Movement is her middle name. In chapter 7, we explain an exercise routine that will give you all the strength, conditioning, flexibility, and energy you need to live the abundant life.

Obviously this lady burns a lot of calories too. That's the other side to the equation. The virtuous woman eats a healthy diet and serves it to her family as well. Her menu may have been like the nutrition plan we detail for you in chapter 3.

> She is like merchant ships;
> She brings her food from afar.
> She rises also while it is still night,
> And gives food to her household.
>
> Proverbs 31:14–15

In Proverbia's day, a balanced diet didn't come to you as it does today. We have supergrand food centers located every three blocks, and specialty businesses will even deliver groceries to your door! In Proverbia's day, you had to go find the food. Ships would bring exotic fruits and vegetables from all over the known world to the docks and the village marketplace. Salt and spices from other lands were rare and even used as trading commodities instead of money. The virtuous woman in Proverbs seeks out healthy foods for herself and her family, and even gets up while it is still dark to prepare wholesome, homemade recipes.

The results of peppy Proverbia's continual pursuit of health for her loved ones: Her husband, known for his accomplishments, has the strength and ability needed to climb the corporate ladder. He sits at the gates with the elders, a place of leadership in their day. He praises his first-rate wife, saying, "Many daughters have done nobly, but you excel them all" (Prov. 31:29).

Proverbia's children also rise up and call her blessed. She's been a busy mom, spending much of her energy on them, actively involved, and looking well to the ways of her household. We don't want our children feeling ashamed of the way we look or act (for instance, rising up and calling us "Chicken Arms" on occasion!), hating the things we say (note Ms. Perfect rules her tongue with wisdom and kindness), or lamenting the way we care for them as mothers. Wouldn't you love to see your teenage son get enough ambition to rise up from the couch and praise you? "Right on, Mom! You're cool!" What a blessing!

But the best reward for right living is the way Proverbia feels about herself. This cheerful, optimistic woman glows with confidence. She's an accomplished woman ("Let her works praise her in the gates," v. 31). She dresses like a queen. The garments that cover her fit body are made from the finest materials, rich in fabric and color. More importantly, strength and dignity clothe her soul. The virtuous woman smiles at the future, according to Scripture.

True Confessions from Cynthia

Trust me, when I am out of shape, I don't smile at the future. I dread the events that lie ahead because I know I don't look my best. I don't feel like myself either. For instance, our publisher called us unexpectedly to arrange the photo shoot for the covers of *The Beautiful Balance* and *The Healthy Balance*. "We need to do the photo shoots *now!*" we were told. Unfortunately this was January, just after Christmas. Research shows that the average person gains an average of seven pounds over the holidays. But I guess I'm not average. I can say I'm above average because I gained more weight than most. My holidays started on November 1 (when I finished this book and started celebrating) and abruptly ended when I got the aforementioned phone call.

I hate to admit it, but fat happens. I had fallen off the *Healthy Balance* wagon. Guzzled eggnog without shame and munched feverishly on goodies I hadn't eaten in years. The only exercise I got was lifting my fork to my mouth. The imbalance showed up around the midline. I won't admit what department I resorted to in order to find a top that matched my jogging pants and Charity's outfit when we were shopping for outfits for the photoshoot for one of our book covers. (Let's just say I didn't want to wait the nine months to fill it out. Call 1-800-REDUCE today!) Proverbia dressed like a queen; I was dressing like an expectant mother. You can bet I cut the tag out of that sweater! (Ever done that?)

At the photo shoot, I solved the problem of not looking my best by always shoving Charity in front of me in the picture. (This works too, sisters. Always stand in the back! You appear smaller that way—or smart and studious, all brain!) I consoled myself that I still had the beauty of Christ to offer my readers. Sniff, sniff. That's what this series is all about, after all—that you can develop your soul in such a way that it satisfies you, attracts others, pleases your Creator, and impacts for eternity. But I wanted to make a little impact now by looking my best. I know that the packaging my soul comes in is important too. I couldn't relate to Proverbia at all during this time of my life. But slumps can be the very catalysts we need to propel us to greatness. After the fact, I climbed back onto the *Healthy Balance* wagon and worked hard to get in shape again. And so can you.

Whom do you relate to, me or Proverbia? Whom would you rather relate to? Would you like to smile at the future too?

Does this picture of the beautifully and healthfully balanced woman excite you? Someday, when you graduate to heaven, would you like this Proverbs epitaph to be read about you? We would! And we hope you would too. We are taking every measure here and now to become the balanced women that God created us to be. Want to come along on the journey? It begins with a single step called Desire. Read chapter 2 to discover the mountain I climbed to gain the health and vitality that every woman wants.

2

My Personal Journey to Wellness

Cynthia's Story

I t was nearly noon when Dr. Thompson, a diagnostician, left the exam room to determine my diagnosis. While he was out I sat on the hard table, ignoring my grumbling stomach. I chewed a fingernail nervously, and with my other hand, I clutched the flimsy paper robe as though it was my last piece of dignity. This physician was not the first I had seen. For months I had endured test after test with doctor after doctor, trying to uncover the reason for my failing health. This time I hoped to get an answer.

Dr. Thompson breezed back into the room. "Lupus," he pronounced matter-of-factly in a voice as cold as the exam room. "Although all your tests aren't conclusive for it, I'm giving you a tentative diagnosis of lupus erythematosus."

My heart fell. Systemic lupus is an incurable disease that causes the body's immune system to attack its own organs.

I knew it was something horrible, I thought. Since college, I had suffered with increasingly poor health. Before that time, I seemed healthy enough: a runner who logged up to fifteen miles a day! But during my senior year in high school, my health—both physical and mental—began to deteriorate. As a freshman in Bible college, my undiagnosed illness forced me to return home midyear. Multiple symptoms like low-grade fever, sore throat, aching muscles, and depression led my doctor to believe I had contracted mononucleosis. (Mono is famous as "the kissing disease" because of its communicability. I swear the only guy I had kissed in my life is now my husband—and he's quite healthy, thank you!)

The ups and downs continued in my early marriage and childbirth days. But even after our first two children (Charity and Chad), I had always gained back my health as soon as I returned to my running program. However, after the birth of our third child, Carly, I collapsed and nearly died. Toxemia, a toxic blood condition that can occur during pregnancy, plagued me in my last few months. I was bedridden the year after the baby's birth as the disease affected every body system, even my brain. Some of my symptoms were:

headaches and brain symptoms (see specifics below)

blurred vision, "roaring ears"

inflammation in my head and spine

joint and muscle pain, aching all over

pleurisy and pain in my lungs, asthma attacks

systemic allergies to foods, chemicals, and other substances

irregular heartbeat and chest pain

bowel irregularities (diarrhea, constipation, bloating)

vascular inflammation, including bursting veins

numbness and tingling

afternoon low-grade fevers
sore throat and swollen glands
chronic fatigue and weakness
repeated vaginal yeast infections
bladder infections
PMS

That's enough misery for one chapter, but you get the idea. When I say "sick from head to toe," I mean it! Incapacitated with excruciating pain and severe weakness, I was unable to maintain my normal routine. My mother and maternal grandmother moved in, taking over my roles of homemaker and mom. The only responsibilities I continued were reading a daily Bible story to my children and home-schooling them, things I could do from my bed.

Following Peter's Damp Footsteps

When I was alone, it wasn't only the pain that kept me awake. Fear became my frequent bedfellow. He wrapped his sticky tentacles around me, squeezing until I was breathless with panic. I worried he would pull me under. I felt like Jesus' disciple out walking on the Sea of Galilee. Like Peter, I couldn't seem to stay above water! Looking around at the stormy waves of circumstances threatening to engulf me, I'd begin to sink into a black sea of despair.

During these times, I cried out to the Lord. I had always had confidence that he heard me before. But now my prayers were short-circuited. They seemed to hit the ceiling and fall back down to me. *Why can't I break through?* I'd wonder. *Is God listening? Does he care? Won't he help me?*

Well-meaning friends increased my discouragement by minimizing my suffering and offering platitudes. They became impatient with my illness. "You should be well by now," they reprimanded.

I kept my mouth shut, but thought, *Don't they realize that I am more tired of this illness than they are?*

One friend whispered to another, "God is chastening her for being out of his will."

When her words got back to me, the Holy Spirit gave me reassurance. *That's not true!* I cried to myself. The year before disease struck me down, I was closer to God than I've ever been, obeying him carefully. *They just don't realize that there are three purposes that God has for allowing illness in a believer's life. To take them home in death, to purify their lives, or to bring glory to himself...*

I thought of Job—no one suffered like that poor saint. Job's suffering brought great glory to God. He's been an example of perseverance ever since. Job had everything taken from him—his health, his livelihood, his children and servants—everything, that is, except a nagging wife and some judgmental friends. Job's buddies didn't understand his suffering either. They didn't see the spiritual work that God was perfecting under the surface. Like a farmer planting a new crop, God knows it takes weeks and months of growth underground before he can harvest a crop of spiritual fruit. Like my friends, Job's buddies didn't understand the spiritual battle being fought at all times in the heavenlies.

But Jesus understands all of this. His suffering on earth was also misunderstood. People even thought his death for our sake was the judgment of God.

Yet it was *our* grief he bore, *our* sorrows that weighed him down. And we thought his troubles were a punishment from God, for his *own* sins! But he was wounded and bruised for *our* sins. He was beaten that we might have peace; he was lashed—and we were healed!

Isaiah 53:4–5 TLB, emphasis added

No one understands like Jesus. However, one bit of advice my friends offered was true. "Simply trust God, Cindy," they counseled. "He's with you in this."

Of course, they were right. But during a journey through the Valley of the Shadow, trusting is not simple. It's important, but not easy. There were times in those months, as my illness progressed and my pain continued, that my desperation led to thoughts of suicide. It was only when I focused on Christ that I had hope for my future. I wrote this in my journal:

Right now, I'm limping through the valley of the shadow of Death. No denying it. This valley is a terrifying place. Darkness. Shadows. Uncertainty. Danger lurking around every corner.

I'm so thankful I have a traveling companion. Strong and capable, he knows the way out of this place.

Pastor Charles Stanley of Atlanta says that the Christian isn't stuck in the valley.

"He's on his way somewhere!" Dr. Stanley assures his radio listeners. "Off to the next glorious step in God's plan for his life." The next step—whether it's heaven, or a new, deeper level of daily life.

"Focus on the destination," Pastor Stanley advises, "not on the circumstances of the journey."

Right now I need to focus on the One who is my escort. Jesus is an expert Guide and Bodyguard. I can *trust him for each step. Like my frightened two-year-old, I grip my companion's hand, trusting him to lead me out. When the valley grows the darkest, I cling to him. His rod and his staff, they comfort me. On the journey, he meets all of my needs, including the grace to see me through. I don't want to give up before I reach the Promised Land. Pastor Stanley guarantees that if I give up, I say that he that is in the world is greater than the One in me.*

It's saying that God is faithful most of the time but not all of the time.

It's proving that I can't put all my weight on him.

I'm relying on my own strength, not his.

God wants to do a miracle in my life . . . if I can just hang on. He's going to do something great in his perfect timing, in his way. And in his strength, I can see this thing through!

"Lord, be a lamp to my feet," I prayed. "Light my path out of this dark valley. Lead me on to your place of peace." My illness caused many brain symptoms:

excruciating headaches that wouldn't let up, migraines

nerve swelling and inflammatory pain in my head and spine

brain fog (If you've had it, you understand this!)

memory loss (Sometimes I wouldn't recognize people I'd known for years, and usually couldn't remember their names!)

mental confusion (The worst. Most days, my brain felt like the static on "snow channels" between networks! Confusing thoughts tortured me. I had to give up driving—I couldn't find my way to routine locations because I would get confused. Shopping was awful. One time I had a hard time counting to four!)

suicidal depression some days (I was in a black tunnel and could see no light).

Finding Hope

In my muddled mental state, I flipped through my Bible to Psalms. I noticed that King David experienced similar emotions when coping with many illnesses during his lifetime. Sometimes it even seemed as if God was not listening. In Psalms, he pleaded with God:

> Lord, hear my prayer! Listen to my plea! Don't turn away from me in this time of my distress. Bend down your ear and give me speedy answers, for my days disappear like smoke. My health is broken and my heart is sick.
>
> Psalm 102:1–4 TLB

> But O my soul, don't be discouraged. Don't be upset. Expect God to act! For I know that I shall again have plenty of reason to praise him for all that he will do. He is my help! He is my God!
>
> Psalm 42:11 TLB

Bypassing my troubled mind, the Spirit spoke to my spirit, and I was comforted. I began to study the Book of Psalms for consolation and the Old Testament for hope. I found many biblical stories that demonstrated how God miraculously worked in the lives of ancient believers. For instance, he saved the Hebrew boys who refused to worship the golden statue. Now there was a fiery trial! Yet they trusted God throughout it. And the Lord was with them in the heat of it. He rescued them from the flaming furnace so completely that they didn't even smell like smoke! And the stories continued . . .

What mercy, faithfulness, and power God revealed to those saints through mighty miracles! As I studied, I discovered who the changeless, almighty God is. He's the same today as he was then. I became assured that he would be with me, as he was with those before me, in all his greatness.

During my sick period (this flare-up lasted five years), the "rubber met the road" regarding my faith. I had always been such a strong Christian, but now I felt so weak and my faith seemed so small. I had to fall down on my knees many times a day to beg his strength and grace to see me through the next few moments. I learned two lessons that assisted me in my journey through illness and then through life: to trust God, no matter what, and to always obey him. "Trust and obey, for there's no other way, to be happy in Jesus," the old hymn says. Peter benefited from a similar education while he was out on the lake. I could relate to his frightening experience as the waves crashed against him.

Crash! Sickness.

Crash! Pain.

Crash! Depression.

Crash! Confusion.

Crash! Uncertain future.

Panic! I'm going under for the third time . . .

Just before Peter plunged completely under, he remembered the Savior and cried, "Lord, save me!"

And Jesus did: "And immediately Jesus stretched out His hand and caught him, and said to him, 'O you of little faith, why did you doubt?'" (Matt. 14:31 NKJV). The Lord gently lifted Peter above the crashing waves into safety.

Then I remembered too. . . . I looked up into the most caring, understanding eyes I'd ever seen. I grasped a gentle, outstretched hand that pulled me up with surprising power. I was safe.

I could depend on the Lord to work illness out for my good and for his glory. I thought of Job again, who had suffered much more than I. Job's trial increased his knowledge of God and helped him worship the Lord in a greater way. This saint's faithfulness brought much praise to the Creator. I determined that my life would do the same.

Days in bed provided me with hours to spend with Christ, a luxury in a house full of children. Pain brought opportunities to trust him more. Unpredictable health taught me to depend on Jesus moment by moment. I ordered Pastor John Hagee's Healing Scripture tapes (see resources on p. 251) and began listening to them every day. Fear was transformed into faith through the truth of God's Word. I grew excited to see how God was going to work. My experience became one of joy and peace . . . and I'm so glad this happened while I was still in the midst of my misery. It showed me that Jesus is truly all I need. However, I kept praying to be healed. After all, it was an unselfish prayer: I had three little children (later five) to raise for the Lord! But months went by, and doctor after doctor released me. Discouraged and frustrated, they couldn't find a cause or a remedy for my disabling condition. I began asking the all-knowing God to reveal what my illness was and how I could get well. I claimed Psalm 32:8 where God says, "I will instruct you . . .

and guide you along the best pathway for your life; I will advise you and watch your progress" (TLB).

"I'm trusting you for answers, Lord," I prayed. "I want you to watch *my* progress!"

My Answer Arrives by U.S. Mail

A year after my "tentative" diagnosis of lupus, an answer to my prayers arrived in the mailbox. My aunt Sharon had spotted a magazine headline as she walked through an airport terminal. "The Missing Diagnosis," read the big, bold type.[1] She picked up the article and began to read.

"That's Cindy!" she exclaimed, so she hurried to the post office.

After reading the piece written by Alabama physician Dr. C. Orian Truss (author of a book entitled *The Missing Diagnosis*), I got excited myself. He was describing me and my symptoms! But I needed to support my newfound belief with research if I was to gain the cooperation of my latest doctor. Still too sick to go out, I sent my Grandmother Garnette to the university library to copy hundreds of medical articles on the subject. Through study, I discovered that years on a lousy diet (junk foods and lots of sugar) had destroyed my immune system. This poor diet, low immunity, and repeated antibiotics allowed an overgrowth of a fungus called *Candida albicans*. Toxins released by the accumulating candida caused many of my miseries, including headaches and other brain symptoms. The colonized yeast had burrowed into many areas of my body, especially my intestines, creating small holes that allowed particles of undigested foods to pass into my bloodstream. As a result, I developed severe food and chemical allergies. The infection and allergies caused my immune system to go into "attack mode," and my autoimmune tendencies flared up (my family has a history of lupus and similar diseases). No wonder I was so sick! After thorough research, I headed to my doctor's office.

"I'm plagued by a systemic candida infection," I explained to my physician, Dr. Malan, a wonderful California physician who truly desires to help his patients. He was almost desperate to find a cure for my illness, but he knew nothing about this condition (which is true of many doctors even today, eighteen years later). Undaunted, I continued. "Here's the medication I need to take," I said, scribbling out my own prescription on his pad.

A powerful antifungal drug called ketoconazole was necessary to kill the candida, which actually live in everyone but grow out of control under certain conditions. (Chapter 6 lists a variety of ways to battle a candida outbreak, including some new medications and lifestyle changes.) Dr. Malan quickly added his signature to my prescription, for which I'll be forever grateful.

That day my life changed. I committed myself to a very strict diet, and within four days my symptoms began to improve. Three weeks after my candida diagnosis, I was privileged to be a guest at a medical conference in San Francisco. The subject: candidiasis, or systemic yeast infections. Physicians were just learning about this illness. At the convention, medical professionals discussed how to diagnose and treat the condition. One report caught my attention: A survey had shown that one in three Americans have a candida problem in varying degrees. This was no surprise, as our normal American diet with its sugary cereals and treats, sodas, French fries and chips, white bread and starches, all contribute to yeast overgrowth. In addition, we eat few foods that build our immune systems, which fight off all diseases from candida to cancer. Other circumstances that predispose a patient to yeast infection are hormone-related conditions (the Pill, multiple pregnancies, and the like), frequent antibiotic use, steroid treatment, and diseases like diabetes and HIV infection.

As Charity and I have traveled around the United States speaking at various churches, conferences, and camps, we've met many Christians with a variety of health problems. So many of us are "sick and tired of being sick and tired" all the time! What kind of a temple can we offer the Holy Spirit if we are run-down and in need of restoration? How can God use us effectively when all we want to do is crawl back into bed as soon as the alarm goes off each morning? We have an enemy who would like to keep us down and out. It's time we told him "where to go" (it's really okay to do so—that's his ultimate destination anyway!), and reclaim the good health God gave most of us at birth. The "cure" for candida (and many other complaints in our country) is so easy—and yet so hard. It takes commitment.

Falling off the Wagon

In the pages that follow, Charity and I outline a plan to heal and renew your body and soul. The *Healthy Balance* program, as we call it, because the plan encompasses the whole person, will take a commitment too. But the benefits of a balanced lifestyle can't be measured by earthly yardsticks. In time, as I committed myself to this healthy diet and lifestyle, my condition improved. However, not a day went by that I didn't have some pain or annoying symptoms. I just learned to live with them, relishing the fact that I was on my feet and so much better than I had been. I enjoyed my children, teaching them at home, resumed my writing ministry, and served in my church. Life was full. I began to enjoy life too much, however, falling off my diet more often than I care to admit.

I didn't realize that the next crash was just around the corner . . .

Our fifth child nearly died at birth from severe RH-incompatibility (unrelated to my health problems). For weeks, my husband and I spent our days and nights at the hospital. For months, I cared for my son while neglecting my own body. I ate thoughtlessly, never truly rested, and didn't fortify my body or relieve my stress through exercise. The burden of caring for a sick newborn and four other children, besides continuing my position on staff of a large church, proved to be too much. As our son recovered, I fell apart. My candida and autoimmune symptoms returned with an unparalleled severity. I was bedridden again, unable to care for myself, let alone my family. I couldn't understand why God had allowed another painful interruption in my life and especially in my service for him.

God is big enough to weather our "Why?" As I sought him for an answer, I remembered that he had always been faithful to me before. The Lord continually provided everything I needed through three previous flare-ups. He had promised to be with me always. This time I trusted the character of God.

In my quiet times, the Lord showed me that with each valley he led me through, my faith increased and my ministry deepened. I learned compassion for other sufferers and developed a heart to serve them. My painful trial exposed my weakness. Again I was in that familiar position many times a day where I had to fall to my knees and beg for mercy to survive the next few minutes. With God's help,

I realized that this is exactly where he wants me—on my knees. Totally dependent on him. The Lord has promised to provide everything I need to live a life for his glory: "My grace is sufficient for you, for my power is made perfect in weakness" (2 Cor. 12:9 NIV).

I still don't like pain, but this verse helps me appreciate it in a new way. When others see the amazing things that God is doing in and through my life, they recognize them as his accomplishments. He receives the praise.

With my health problems, my life could have amounted to so much of nothing—days, weeks, and even years in bed. But through the Lord's intervention, Ephesians 3:20 has become a reality for me. I have made it my life verse.

> "Now to him who is able to do immeasurably more than all we ask or imagine, according to his power that is at work within us, to him be glory."
>
> Ephesians 3:20–21 NIV

I now have a beautiful Christian family (a husband, five children, and a son-in-law who love the Lord); a writing ministry that has touched millions of lives; a career in the health field; and the joy of having led many people to salvation in Christ. But best of all, I've come to know God in a way I never could have without my valley experiences. I can know his presence, peace, and power in spite of pain and disease.

Lessons Learned for Good

These spiritual blessings would be enough, certainly. But God chose to heal my illness too. During my last flare-up, I realized that I had a chronic condition—I would live with it the rest of my life. That meant that even when I feel better, I don't go off the diet (or at least don't cheat too much too often!). I continue a healthy lifestyle—or else! In the ensuing chapters of *The Healthy Balance,* Charity and I reveal everything we have gleaned from years of research, personal experience, interviews with physicians, and stories from others. I'm so thankful for all that my illness has taught me. I've learned so much, both for the body and the soul, and have been able to help hundreds of sick people. And through this book and those to come (praise God!), I am able to share these liberating truths with thousands. I can offer the testimony that my health today (as I hover dangerously near fifty) is better than it was at twenty. I couldn't have said this nine years ago, but life is beautiful! And I wouldn't have said this nine years ago, but . . . I hope I live to ninety-seven! I have the strength, energy, and health now to do all that God has called me to do, and to actually enjoy doing it! Health and happiness can be the next chapter in your life too!

3

Healthy Balance Foods
for Body and Soul

Are you the picture of health, and do you want to stay that way? Or perhaps you too are sick and tired of being sick and tired. Has your doctor recently given you a diagnosis that scares the life out of you? No matter which question you answered or which author you relate to—Charity's health maintenance or Cynthia's health renewal—this chapter will provide you with the necessary information for fantastic health. Nutritional healing is the cutting edge of medicine today. Dr. Linda Page claims that we can "heal with every meal." But the value of healing foods is not a new idea. In the fifth century B.C., Hippocrates, the father of medicine, said, "Let your food be your medicine and your medicine be your food."

Pliny the Elder, in his book *Natural Healing,* claimed that "it would be a long task to make a list of all the praises of cabbage." Nevertheless, he listed eighty-seven medicinal uses for the common garden vegetable. And the Chinese, one of the world's oldest civilizations, have never drawn a distinction between food and medicine, according to Chinese writer Lin Yutang.

Down through the centuries, people had an innate sense of what was good for them. Perhaps this knowledge was passed from generation to generation, originating with Adam and Eve. In the beginning, God created the world and every good thing in it. According to Genesis 1 and 2, he planted a garden and placed the first man and woman there. Then God said, "Behold, I have given you every plant yielding seed that is on the surface of all the earth, and every tree which has fruit yielding seed; *it shall be food for you*" (Gen. 1:29, emphasis added).

> Tell me what you eat and I will tell you what you are.
>
> Anthelme Brillat-Savarin (1755–1826)

Good nutrition for all creatures included plant foods fresh from the earth that had produced them. The Creator knew the wholesome edibles that would best provide abundant health for his flesh-and-blood creations. Later, after the flood, God initiated meat consumption. Perhaps his knowledge that the altered earth would no longer grow sufficient vegetation brought about this new rule. We don't know. But God said, "*Every moving thing that is alive shall be food for you; I give all* to you, as I gave the green plant" (Gen. 9:3, emphasis added). Our food is one of God's gifts to his creation, and in that moment, the Creator redefined his healthy diet plan for humankind: live foods from plants and flesh foods from anything that moved.

Since then, humans have been predominately hunter-gatherers. They've foraged for fruits and vegetables and eaten the wild game they killed. And they got plenty of exercise chasing around that night's dinner! When civilized societies began to grow grain and other crops, they demonstrated the same symptoms of ill health that plague Americans today. Excavation of Egypt's tombs has revealed corpses who succumbed to familiar diseases: heart disease, diabetes, strokes, and obesity. Remember the Bible story of Jacob's family traveling to Egypt to buy grain during a famine? Jacob's own son, Joseph, had recommended that Pharaoh stockpile surplus grain for the coming famine. In biblical times, the mighty Nile civilization luxuriated in an abundance similar to that which the United States enjoys today. The Egyptians also suffered from equivalent ailments. Our modern Western diet of white flour, sugar, and fried or processed foods replaced meats and fresh plant foods. Sodas full of chemicals but no nutrition have been substituted for water and healthy juices. Should we be surprised that most of us don't enjoy a high-quality life, when we have such a low-quality diet?

> Healthy Balance
> secret #1:
> *Learn to love
> live foods!*

After years of study, we can sum up our diet and nutrition advice in a nutshell (pun intended—sorry!). We offer seven secrets to living a healthy balanced life. Our first secret for the *Healthy Balance* plan: *Learn to love live foods!*

Live foods? We're talking plants here, not the live dinner the hunters of old chased around. (Gross! Vegetarianism sounds appealing with that thought!)

Live plant foods have enzymes, protein molecules that initiate every biochemical reaction in the body. Called the "sparks of life," enzymes make all of our brain and body functions possible. Although our bodies do make some enzymes, most of these essential catalysts come from food. The food must be raw, however, as heat, beginning at 102 degrees, destroys enzymes. Cooked food is dead food. There are no enzymes in it, and dead food is not what we need to sustain life as God planned it. Eating cooked and processed foods only puts a burden on the pancreas. The real job of the pancreas is to produce insulin and special enzymes to keep tropoblastic cancer cells under control. After a meal of completely cooked food, this organ has to also produce enzymes for digestion that should already be in the food. After years of eating this way, the pancreas will swell to several times its normal size. In time it will be unable to do its job, affecting other organs and the immune system. Thus begins the downward spiral into ill health.

Fresh fruits and vegetables are perfect for today's lifestyle concerns.

Worried about weight? Packed with life-giving vitamins and minerals, fruits and vegetables are fat-free or very low fat.

Always in a hurry? With no preparation time required, fruits and veggies are nature's original fast food, quick to grab on the go.

Embracing environmental causes? Whole foods don't litter the landscape (except for biodegradable peels, they leave no wrappers behind).

Bored with your diet? In a penny pinch? In industrialized nations, a variety of produce from the everyday apple to the exotic lychee fruit is widely available and affordable at the neighborhood grocery.

News Flash! Science Agrees with God

The always conservative National Institutes of Health has issued guidelines for a new way of eating. Their latest trend is to push vegetables and fruits, something that health-conscious individuals have always done. The NIH has a motto to follow: 5 a day for better health. Half of all Americans consume only a single serving of fruits or vegetables a day.[1] Amazingly, 10 percent of Americans eat no produce at all. Another 10 percent eat five or fewer fruits and vegetables a day. Market surveys reveal what those five foods are. Americans repeatedly purchase iceberg lettuce, tomatoes (in sauces and ketchup), potatoes (including fries and other frozen products), bananas, and oranges (as juice). One researcher stated, "If it wasn't for the French fry, most Americans would have scurvy."[2]

This malnutrition is occurring in the land of plenty. Americans' food choices are appalling and fall far short of God's original plan and even the low NIH resolution. In reality, the body's need for plant life nutrition far exceeds even their recommendations.

Researchers have found that a person will thrive when he or she ingests at least nine servings of fruits and vegetables each day. (If that sounds like a system overload, remember that a serving is only a half cup. And nine servings is only three a meal!) Variety is not only the spice of life, it's also essential for good health. God knew this and created for our consumption over 150,000 edible plant species. Talk about temptations to overeat! Hunter-gatherer populations in remote locations like New Guinea eat more than eight hundred types of plant foods. You can see why Americans are bored with their diet—we eat the same colorless meals over and over. Our daily diet is *overwhelmed* with calories and *underwhelmed* with nutrition. Perhaps that's why one in two Americans is overweight or clinically obese—and still not satisfied. Our culture's temptations are fast-food joints on every corner offering tasty foods loaded with calories, fats, sugars, and chemicals, but empty of any nutrition—dead foods that will tax and burden the body. Now that we know the truth, it's time Americans took charge of their diet. Don't let foods control you. Use foods for your edification as God intended. In the following pages, we'll explain how.

The New Old Idea

I (Cynthia) discovered the value of fresh, live foods back in 1985. During recovery from my serious candida infection and autoimmune flare-up, I stumbled upon a book entitled *The Candida Albicans Yeast-Free Cookbook,* originally published in 1985 by Pat Connolly and The Price-Pottenger Nutrition Foundation. This nutritional program was instrumental in restoring my health. Weston Price, D.D.S., a nutritional pioneer who observed eating patterns of healthy people throughout remote areas of the world, first formulated a healing program in the 1920s.

> Your food shall be your remedy. Let food be your medicine and let medicine be your food.
>
> Hippocrates, Greek physician, 5th century B.C.

Dr. Price found that these robust groups derived their nutrition from whole foods native to their habitat. Another dentist, Dr. Melvin Page, who studied the Price research, applied these findings to his patients. He advised them to also avoid all refined foods, especially sugar. (Refined sugar has been available only since the 1600s.) Through precise laboratory analyses, Dr. Page discovered that when patients ate sugar and other refined foods, their blood chemistries became abnormal. As soon as they adopted a diet of fresh vegetables, whole grains, and protein, their blood chemistries shifted back to normal.

These dentists, Dr. Price and Dr. Page, along with dentist and nutritionist Dr. Bruce Pacetti, developed an eating plan that incorporated their research findings. Their diet supersedes the latest recommendations of the NIH. Imagine your plate at your next meal filled with foods mirroring every color of the rainbow. This is the easy solution that Doctors Price, Page, and Pacetti offer to ensure that you get the necessary nutrients, enzymes, and phytochemicals that your body needs for good health. We want to present to you a new diet based on old, tested principles. After our research, we've made some important additions and simplifications to the concepts. We call our plan *The Healthy Balance.* In it, you will get all the nutrition you need for good health for both body and soul.

Back to Egypt

Growing up, you were taught the four basic food groups: protein, starches, dairy, produce. That concept became as extinct as the dinosaurs. The USDA offered us the Food Guide Pyramid. This definitely changed our minds about what was needed by the human body for good health. As research continued, the pyramid evolved.

We'd like to offer the *Healthy Balance* pyramid to give you a visual illustration of the plan. On our nutritional program, you'll eat lots of fresh fruits and vegetables, lean meats, poultry, fish, eggs, whole grains and legumes, nonfat dairy, especially yogurt, good oils and butter, and nuts and seeds. We will offer suggestions for those who want to eat only plant foods. The healthy foods on the *Healthy Balance* plan will provide you with every nutrient known to science and also some that haven't been discovered yet. Research is revealing more and more micronutrients that we didn't even know existed. But God did; he created them! And by eating the way he planned, we fulfill our bodies' requirements, even when we don't have full knowledge of the process. Supplements aren't substitutes for a healthy diet. But the hurried, haphazard eating in our hectic world begs for supplementation. Along with our eating plan, take a daily basic vitamin/mineral pill with at least the minimums of

Vitamin A, B complex, C, D, E, selenium, calcium, iron, zinc, and other essential minerals.

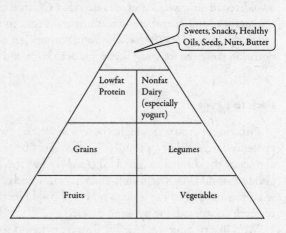

Sweets, Snacks, Healthy Oils, Seeds, Nuts, Butter

Lowfat Protein

Nonfat Dairy (especially yogurt)

Grains

Legumes

Fruits

Vegetables

God's Multivitamins for the Soul

Spiritually we have some nutrients that are essential for the health of our souls:

Vitamin A is physically necessary for healthy skin. Retin-A is a powerful dose of this vitamin that, when applied to skin, heals and restores its youthful appearance. Spiritually, we have something like our skin. It's called the flesh. We need to apply the Holy Spirit's control to resist the desires of the flesh. "But I say, walk by the Spirit, and you will not carry out the desire of the flesh" (Gal. 5:16).

Vitamin B gives us physical energy. The Holy Spirit energizes us to serve Christ with our bodies, minds, and spirits.

Vitamin C fortifies our immune system against attacks from outside agents like viruses, bacteria, and parasites. Putting on the full armor of God guards us from attacks by the enemy of our souls.

Vitamin D, needed for bone health, comes from the sun. Everything we need for robust living comes from the Son, Jesus Christ. "Abide in Me," he tells us. "I am the vine, you are the branches; he who abides in Me and I in him, he bears much fruit; for apart from Me you can do nothing" (John 15:4–5).

Vitamin E protects the heart. Proverbs 4:23 warns us, "Above all else, guard your heart, for it affects everything you do" (NLT).

Iron-enriched bread. We need iron for strength. Many baked goods are fortified with this mineral. God's Word is our daily bread in life. Daily intake of Scripture will give us all the strength necessary to live the Christian life abundantly.

Salt, in the right amount, is an essential element for physical health. Salt is so important that in biblical times it was used as money! That's how valued it was. Jesus calls us "the salt of the earth." Too much of a good thing can be irritating. But in just the right amounts, our saltiness preserves righteousness and creates a thirst for Jesus Christ. And we are very valuable to our Lord!

H_2O. Speaking of thirst . . . water is the most critical substance of all for health. A human can survive weeks without food. Got water? No? You're history! You will only live a few days without this all-important liquid. Water constitutes 90 percent of your blood, 75 percent of your brain and muscles, 20 percent of your body fat, and 22 percent of your bone. It is needed for all bodily functions including transporting nutrients and oxygen around your body, eliminating waste, maintaining body temperature, lubricating joints, cushioning organs and tissues, keeping skin moisturized, and many other things. Our bodies need eight to ten cups of pure water a day.

For our soul, Jesus is "living water." He is the one who is crucial to our spiritual health. He is necessary for our very lives, and we can't survive a day without him. Without Jesus, we become spiritually dehydrated. With him, however, we will know abundant life and true satisfaction. He told the woman at the well,

"Whoever drinks of the water that I will give him shall never thirst; but the water that I will give him will become in him a well of water springing up to eternal life."

John 4:14

"If anyone is thirsty, let him come to Me and drink. He who believes in Me, as the Scripture said, 'From his innermost being will flow rivers of living water.'" But this He spoke of the Spirit, whom those who believed in Him were to receive."

John 7:37–39

The *Healthy Balance* Plan

Your *Healthy Balance* meals should center around fruits and vegetables, not the meat or entree, as is common in America. A man from Europe once told us, "In the United

States, one person's steak would make a family's dinner in my country." You only need to eat about 3 ounces (oz) of protein (the size of a deck of cards) per meal to satisfy your daily protein requirement. The popular and healthful Mediterranean Diet features lots of plant foods, with meat and pasta as condiments.

With a *Healthy Balance* plate, your aim is color. You can even make it a game to see how many colors you can incorporate into each meal, into each day. You can ask family members, "Did you eat your colors today?" or "How many colors did you eat at dinner?"

The pigment of each vegetable and fruit is important, providing unique benefits to your body. Your *Healthy Balance* day should include portions from these valuable food groups: a complete protein; a grain and legume (which combined can create a complete protein); nonfat dairy, especially yogurt; healthy oils, seeds, and nuts; and ten servings of vegetables and fruits in these colors: red, purple, orange, yellow, green, white-green, and a green leafy vegetable. If this sounds like a lot of food, you only need to eat small portions to make sure you are getting proper nutrients. The ideal "balanced plate" will leave you feeling light and comfortable. Need to lose some extra pounds? This just might be the ticket to rid yourself of excess fat and improve your health in the same process!

Protein for your meal can be the low-fat white meat of poultry, fish or seafood, eggs, or soy protein. Enjoy lean pieces of red meat or pork only once in a while. If you eat grains and legumes at the same meal, they combine into a complete protein with all the amino acids your body requires.

The grains and legumes include whole unprocessed grains like long-grain brown rice, whole oats, corn or whole wheat products, and any kind of dry beans cooked without fat. (You can eat a small amount of these at each meal or save your high-carbs to eat at one sitting.)

The red group includes tomatoes and tomato products, red peppers, watermelon, strawberries, cherries, red apples, and pink grapefruit.

Purple plants are grapes and grape juice, red cabbage, blackberries, blueberries, raisins, beets, prunes, plums, cranberries, eggplant, and red wine.

The orange category is filled with foods like pumpkin, carrots, winter squash, sweet potatoes, mangoes, apricots, oranges and orange juice, tangerines, and cantaloupes.

For yellow produce, look for corn, crookneck squash, yellow grapefruit, yellow peppers, peaches, lemons, limes, papayas, pineapples, and nectarines.

The all-important green category is comprised of green peas and beans, broccoli, brussel sprouts, avocados, green peppers, cabbage and Chinese cabbage, and kiwi.

White-green edibles include onion and garlic, cauliflower, turnips, radishes, celery, leeks, asparagus, pears, artichokes, mushrooms, cucumbers, chives, and white wine.

Green leafy vegetables are very important! They are kale, collards, turnip greens, spinach, Swiss chard, mustard greens, bok choy, cabbage, and dark green leafy lettuces.

Dairy products should be nonfat yogurt, milk, buttermilk, and low-fat cheese or cottage cheese. Soy milk or products can replace the dairy ones if allergies exist.

Seeds and nuts are good for snacks but should be eaten in moderation. Also include in the diet 2 tablespoons (Tbs) of healthy oils a day (extra-virgin olive oil, canola, flaxseed, avocado, or a nut oil).

Easy Does It

You may be saying, "The *Healthy Balance* plan is like an old-fashioned recipe. Too many ingredients for my taste!" But it is the variety that provides the nutrients our bodies need. This was proven in a study with rats. Scientists fed one group of rodents a diet of bland, white food. The other group ate their regular rat diet of yellow foods, corn, and the like. The second group thrived, while the white-foods group died within three months! Try to include as much color in your diet as you can. It's actually not difficult to prepare colorful meals once you get used to it.

Eating the *Healthy Balance* way really is addictive. Both of us have periods when we "fall off the nutrition wagon." We eat junk on the run. In no time, though, we are hungering for our wholesome foods. It's so satisfying when we get back on the program of fruits and vegetables, whole grains,

---

Cynthia Shares

The benefits of the *Healthy Balance* diet are quickly apparent and pay off big-time. After only a few months on a strict version of the plan, I was praised by my doctor when my blood tests came back with exemplary results.

"Whatever you're doing, keep it up!" my doctor exclaimed.

Over time I even lost too much weight, and my cholesterol dipped so low that I was forced to use cream on my hot cereal—torture! All this, in spite of smothering my vegetables in butter! But my blood pressure dropped to a low-normal ideal, and my diagnostic tests revealed perfect health.

You can experience the same results with a produce-based, protein-rich diet. In chapter 5, we share easy methods of implementing this health-giving eating plan. You can also try some of our favorite recipes on your family to get them hooked on nutrition!

legumes, yogurt, and protein. We can liken this good food addiction to our souls' need for solid spiritual food. Psalm 34:8 says, "O taste and see that the LORD is good." When we first come to Christ, we are spiritual infants. Babies demand milk and lots of it. The church must be in the "dairy business" for its young believers, giving them what's good for them. They need the milk of the Word—the foundational truths of God's love and forgiveness that are palatable and easily assimilated.

Toss Us a Bone!

But we don't want to stay at the baby food level in our Christianity. It's tempting, we know. Oh, that creamy milk—it goes down so smooth! But we older Christians need some meat to sink our teeth into. Meat can be tough (these truths take some deep thinking, struggling over, and acting on), but the gnawing strengthens our teeth and makes us strong.

We recently bought a honey-colored cocker spaniel puppy. When Spike (as our youngest named him) was tiny, he hungrily lapped up his milk. He craved it, and the liquid food was good for him. Now that Spike is nine months old, he only gets a bit of milk in his bowl as an occasional treat. Instead, we feed him meat and bones to build up his teeth and jaws and to help him grow. Besides, if we don't toss him a bone, Spike chews up everything else to satisfy his crunch cravings!

Aren't we just like that as Christians? We don't feed our spiritual appetites with the spiritual food God prescribes for our nourishment. In our churches, so often we are still offered milk, no matter what our maturity level. On top of that, we fill our souls with the fast food of the world—its movies, music, and entertainment; its money, power, and fame; its values and philosophies; its shallowness and busy activities—and we wonder why we are still hungry inside. We eat more and more junk spiritually and never satisfy our cravings or quench our thirst. Our souls were made for meat—for whole, living spiritual food, not the world's table scraps. We have both experienced this firsthand. We get really busy and don't take the time to eat decent spiritual meals. We survive on spiritual fast food and junk food for several months. A daily devo here, a radio message there, an inspirational movie or two. Then the emptiness in our souls grumbles so loudly it must be fed! The hunger we know is only satisfied through in-depth Bible study. That's why years ago we both took a precept course in inductive Bible study. We've been feasting on the meat of the Word ever since. And just like healthy whole foods, once you get a taste for healthy whole spiritual food, you'll never be content with anything else!

Foods That Cleanse, Foods That Heal

Because I (Cynthia) had a candida problem (an overgrowth of a yeast that feeds on sugar), I ate no fruit during my recovery period. The body can do quite well on vegetables, seeds, nuts, legumes, and proteins. I ate those food groups, plus a small amount of butter and olive oil, for many years. My health improved dramatically! The Price-Pottenger Nutrition Foundation recommends fruit only for special treats.

If natural sugars are no problem for you, add fresh fruit to your diet. These sweet low-fat treats are packed with nutrients and enzymes. You will want to eat more vegetables than fruits, however. A good rule to remember: Fruits are cleansing; vegetables are healing. If you've been eating a lot of junk food, you may want to go on a cleansing program. Watch for our upcoming LifeBalance book, *The Inner Balance for Body and Soul,* that details how to do this. But until it comes out, an easy way to cleanse your system is to eat only fruit for two to three days. Drink lots of pure water. You'll clear out plenty of toxins on this "fruit fast." Try this only if you don't have candida, diabetes, or another condition affected by sugar. Candida sufferers can detox by drinking vegetable juices and eating vegetables, raw or lightly steamed, for several days.

Vegetables are healing and strengthening. They build you up. That's why cancer clinics and other alternative medical centers recommend a diet rich in produce and other live foods. Vitamins, minerals, phytochemicals, and enzymes provide the body with everything it needs to heal itself. Phytochemicals, or "phytonutrients" as they are also called, are compounds that safeguard your genes and DNA, thus protecting and restoring your body's health. Plants get the colors in their skins from absorbing the sun's light. It's this energy that our bodies need so desperately to sustain life. Always eat vegetables carefully washed and unpeeled when possible.

Out with the Old

In 1997, Reader's Digest Association published a valuable book entitled *Foods That Harm, Foods That Heal.* We listed a small number of the good, healing foods. But there are also some foods to stay away from. Don't worry, there are more good than bad. It's just that the bad are so tempting! It's the old "forbidden fruit" problem. Back in Eden, God told Adam and Eve, "You can eat all the plants and fruits in the Garden," then he added, "all except for this one." Where did their eyes instantly shoot? That tree. Which tree were they soon hanging around? That forbidden one, the one food choice that would harm them. The twosome should have stayed as far away from trouble as possible.

The same is true for you as you begin a new diet—get rid of the old troublesome one first. We hate to break the news, but *sugar is trouble*. It stimulates the appetite. People who eat refined, sugary, processed foods consume 25 percent more calories than those who eat natural whole foods. Unfortunately, refined sugar is in everything nowadays, even canned vegetables! And it only takes 1 Tbs of refined sugar to impair the immune system for up to four days. Even the Bible says to control your intake of sweets. "Do you like honey? Don't eat too much of it, or it will make you sick!" Proverbs 25:16 (TLB) warns. Honey may be natural, but it's still sugar in the bloodstream. From experience, I (Cynthia) can attest that too much sugar of any kind will make you sick. And I know you can live without it! Back in 1984, before I compiled the *Healthy Balance* diet, I was a choco-sugar-carb-aholic. I haven't eaten sugar since 1985, and I don't even miss it!

Now, out with the old. . . . Clear your cupboards of anything made with sugar, white flour, packaged mixes, white rice, and other depleted, fattening foods. Peanut butter cookies on the shelf. Potato chips in the cupboard. Lemon meringue pie in the frig. Mocha fudge ice cream in the freezer. Whatever tempts you, out with it! If you can't bear to throw food away (like Cynthia), share it at your next church potluck or youth gathering, or use it up gradually and replace with healthy foods. Wipe out your cupboards, refrigerator, and freezer, then you're ready to go shopping.

In with the new. . . . At the supermarket, shop the outer perimeter of the store. The shelves against the four outside walls are where the fresh, healthier foods are displayed. We know this perimeter well, so we can tell you exactly what you'll find. Grab a cart and follow behind us as we enter New Way Food SuperCenter. Head to the produce section, where you'll spot all the colorful fruits and vegetables we've been raving about. You'll want to pick up the ingredients for a big salad. (If the next few days will be especially busy, healthy salads come prepackaged. Look for the bags with dark, leafy greens, not iceberg lettuce.) Select some veggies for our soup recipe on page 115. You'll also want several other vegetables for dinner side dishes. Keep your "colors" in mind and choose accordingly. And don't forget plenty of onions and garlic! Remember, the Hebrews craved these and were ready to return to Egypt for them. Food without seasoning can be mighty intolerable.

Always choose the freshest, highest quality foods available. Living in America has its advantages! Sometimes we are awed when we walk through a produce section. Look at the abundance God has given our nation. The blessings in America are truly amazing, aren't they? We sometimes breathe a word of thanks right there in the store.

Pick out some tempting fruits for breakfasts and snacking. Bag some lemons and limes for the week. What about an avocado for guacamole after the big game on Friday night? Be sure to stock plenty of seasonings like cayenne, cumin, curry, cinnamon, ginger, garlic powder, and other favorites.

Sometimes the bread display is near the produce. There's nothing wrong with day-old bread either. Just watch for mold. And don't be fooled by packaging or advertising. Content is what you're after! You want whole-grain baked goods with little or no sugar and fat. Corn tortillas should be made with

> When eating fruit, think of the person who planted the tree!

corn or masa, water, and possibly lime. The purer and simpler the ingredients in your food, the healthier you'll be. Learn to read labels. Your health depends on it!

Select some butter in the dairy section, along with plain, acidophilus yogurt. If you like cottage cheese, you can purchase a nonfat variety. The eggs are usually in this section too. Place a dozen or two in your cart, depending on how many mouths you have to feed. Farm eggs are the best but are not always available. In the dairy cooler, there are several options we like: milk with 1 percent fat for drinking and using on cereals, low-fat buttermilk for dressings, and cream for splurging.

In the meat department, select low-fat proteins like chicken, turkey, fresh fish, and soy products. Shellfish is also a good choice. I (Charity) also purchase baby bay shrimp to toss into our salads. Even though my husband says he's a meat-and-potato man, we limit ourselves to one special meat of the week, either beef, lamb, or pork.

Stop and shop in the frozen section. Juices are flash-frozen to retain most of their nutrients. The same is true of vegetables and fruits. We use mostly fresh produce, but women who work away from home may want to fill their freezers with healthy, easy-to-prepare frozen foods. Select a few frozen veggies, some fruits for morning shakes and desserts, and fish fillets. Even some of the TV dinners are nutritious. Read the labels and don't depend on prepared

---

Charity Chats

I usually shop for produce at my local farmer's market once every week or two. Produce is lower priced there than at chain groceries, and it's fresher and cared for better. If your only shopping option is a supermarket, however, you can check the "reduced section" in the produce department. You'll find bags of miscellaneous produce at discounted prices. Most stores put the markdowns out at a certain time of day. Ask your produce manager what time it's done at your store. Keep in mind that store produce is ripe and needs to be refrigerated or eaten promptly.

Recently I bought a bag containing 3 mangoes, 1 pound of grapes, 2 apples, and 1 pound of strawberries for 99 cents. Another 99-cent bag contained 3 yellow peppers, 2 red peppers, a carton of sliced mushrooms, 1 onion, and 3 avocados. We bought our fruit and vegetables for the week for under two dollars!

---

foods too often. To have ever-ready homemade dishes available, career women can prepare the week's meals ahead of time and pop them in the freezer if necessary. One of us (Charity) cooks ahead on the weekend, and the other (Cynthia) cooks ahead on Monday morning (so by the weekend her food has run out and her husband has to take her out to dinner!).

Just a few more aisles and we're done shopping. You'll want to add your favorite dried beans to your basket: pintos, blacks, small whites. Choose several grains too: brown rice, barley, oats, wheat (unless you have an allergy like Cynthia). Your cereals, hot and cold, should also be whole-grain. The healthiest boxed cereals are Shredded Wheat and Grape-Nuts. Wheaties might be the "breakfast of champions," but it's not a healthy, balanced woman's first meal of the day.

Some canned or bottled products are handy in a pinch. Choose spaghetti sauces with little or no sugar. You can also

~~Cynthia Shares~~

A healthy diet doesn't mean a bland one, and an occasional treat can add variety. My favorite yogurts are Mountain High Original and Brown Cow Cream Top Whole Milk Yogurt. Yes, I actually eat the cream on the top as soon as I get home from the store! Once I get rid of that blasted cream, I am left with a low-fat yogurt!

I also keep nonfat canned milk on my shelves to add to hot cereal and coffee. It seems richer. Coffee is a favorite indulgence, and I buy the good stuff like Starbucks or Thanksgiving. I mix coffee beans at the store, different varieties for flavor, and grind them myself.

Caffeine can be addicting, so you have to be careful with your coffee consumption (or you can try decaffeinated). You can even mix your coffee beans half regular and half decaf at the store and grind them together.

purchase whole-grain pastas that are more nutritious than white flour noodles. Salsas are tasty over eggs, meat, and baked potatoes. Low-sodium fat-free chicken broth is good to store for quick soups and other recipes like our Skinny Mashed Potatoes. Canned tuna makes a hurried lunch, and green olives are great chopped into it. Speaking of olives, you'll want extra-virgin olive oil. Olive oil is a healthy oil with monounsaturated fats that are actually good for you in small amounts. Pick up some nonstick butter-flavored spray for pan-broiling meats or scrambling eggs.

Canned, precooked legumes can be tossed into soups and salads for extra protein and vitamins. Fat-free refried beans are good for tostadas and burritos. Low-fat popcorn to microwave or air pop is a good snack choice.

Buy a can of almonds too. If you're on the run and need something quick and nutritious, nothing beats a handful of nuts. But if losing weight is a priority, eat only a serving. They are full of fats. Let the nuts replace your next meat serving. Thin people can munch on nuts all they want. Nuts are packed with vitamins, minerals, monounsaturated fats (good fats that actually lower cholesterol), and antioxidants (age and disease busters).

In the beverage aisle, grab several bottles of mountain spring water if you don't have a purifier. Flavored (but not sweetened) carbonated water is a fun treat. Taste some new types of tea. Have you tried green tea yet? It's the latest rage for getting antioxidants into your body. In China they've been drinking it for years. We use artificial sweeteners to flavor our drinks. We've done extensive research on their effects on health. Some of the research findings over the years were erroneous; on some sweeteners, the jury is still out. Sweet'N Low (saccharin, pink packages) has been around for almost one hundred years and has demonstrated no ill effects on humans. Equal is a newer sweetener made from aspartame (blue packages). There have been some complaints of headaches and allergic reactions with its use. Experiment with it carefully. We use it in moderation, as we do Splenda (sucralose, yellow packages). The beauty of having three choices is that you can alternate them and not get too much of any one type of sweetener. Stevia is also a natural sweetener available from health food stores.

What to Do with All This Food?

Once home, place 1 pound of butter on the counter to soften. (You'll need it for our Balanced Butter recipe in chapter 5.) Choose a cupboard shelf for your canned foods and put them away. Arrange your refrigerator so you know just where everything is. Rinse the greens and lettuces, dry, and refrigerate in storage bags. (Authors' tip: If you clean the produce right away, like we do, you'll be more apt to use it.) Wash the apples, pears, plums, and oranges, then place them in a crystal bowl in the center of your lovely table. Appealing fruits make quick, wholesome snacks.

Wash your produce thoroughly to remove pesticides, dirt, and bacteria. Buy organic if you can afford it. But since organic produce can be very expensive, we are choosy about what we buy at health food stores. The most important produce to purchase organically are leafy vegetables like kale, spinach, collard greens, Swiss chard, cabbage, and lettuces. In research we found that leafy vegetables accumulate the most pesticides, protruding from the ground like they do. Next come plants like broccoli, celery, cauliflower, and apples. We never buy root vegetables like carrots, sweet potatoes, onions, turnips, and beets at pricey organic grocers because they are grown underground. The same goes for produce that we peel, like winter squash, bananas, cucumbers, kiwis, and onions. You can decide what's best for you and your family. Try a farmer's market and ask what pesticides are used, or hopefully not used.

You can make a gentle vegetable wash for your produce. Donald Payne, a manager at S and S Produce health superstore in northern California, created this wash, which is an excellent sterilizer:

Veggie Wash

Boil 2 cups water with 1 teaspoon (tsp) salt for two minutes and cool.

Add 1 cup hydrogen peroxide.

Pour this mixture into 2 gallons of water in a sink or container, and soak produce for two minutes.

Rinse produce well, allow to dry, and refrigerate.

Now, what to do with all this food? We've discovered that keeping soup and salad in the frig, ready-to-eat, keeps us on the *Healthy Balance* eating plan. Follow the recipes in chapter 5. We offer salad recipes on pages 113–15. Prepare that to have ready when hunger strikes. You can make a big pot of nutritious soup with our recipes on pages 117–20. Wonder if you have time for all that chopping? Think of a time waster you could cut out once or twice a week to make your family a healthy soup or crock of beans. Once, we heard an Italian woman who was a guest on a radio health program. She explained that in Europe homemakers go out each morning to buy fresh produce for their daily meals. Then they return home, basket of veggies on their arms. Soon they've whipped up a nourishing soup or stew.

"American women say they have no time for homemade meals," she chided. "But they find time to go to exercise class. They find time to chat on the phone or Internet. They find time to watch television. Let them use that hour to make their families a healthy soup."

Handmade Heart Talks

A food processor or Vita-Mix will speed up chopping-dicing-slicing time. But I (Cynthia) honestly relish my time alone in the kitchen. I listen to Scripture tapes and have "read" through the Bible many times while cooking for my family. A lot of love goes into my meals, while a lot of Love goes into me. By the time we finish dinner, I can honestly say the meal has been good for at least one body and soul—mine!

Alone again in the kitchen? (Have you ever noticed that everyone else takes off when they hear you hard at work at the sink?) Don't feel resentful. Thank God for precious quiet time to think. The Lord has taught me some of his most precious lessons as I was chopping vegetables. While dissecting an onion, he reminds me that he works on me in similar fashion.

How do we peel an onion? Layer by layer. I pull back the top layer of skin (God is removing my fear and lack of faith). Another layer off (there goes my lust and greed). Another layer (my critical attitude). Now we're to the heart of the matter.

Bam! He takes the knife to me (shades of Emeril Lagasse!) and begins to chop, removing the gossip in my life. Bam! God really takes the knife to me—chop, chop, chop—destroying my selfishness. The whole process is quite stinky, and as you know, can bring tears to our eyes.

Sometimes God has to completely crush me, as I do a clove of garlic. He uses circumstances, illness, disappointment, authority figures, and loss to pulverize the last bits of my pride. Then, after he has taken me through the fire (I usually toss the crushed garlic into a saute pan at this point), my essence is released, and I'm palatable and useable.

Although these lessons are sometimes painful, I honestly don't mind the Lord's discipline, do you? And I know he brings every "spiritual spanking" my way out of pure, unconditional love. It is the Lord's kindness that moves us to repentance.

We should treat others in the same loving way. How do you handle an avocado? Carefully and gently because it bruises easily! The Bible admonishes us to handle believers who sin carefully and gently, like we do a piece of fruit. We don't want to bruise them!

"Let us not become boastful," Galatians 5:26 says. Chapter 6:1–3 goes on:

"Brethren, even if anyone is caught in *any* trespass, *you who are spiritual,* restore such a one in a spirit of gentleness; each one looking to yourself, so that you too will not be tempted. Bear one another's burdens, and thereby fulfill the law of Christ. For if anyone thinks he is something when he is nothing, he deceives himself" (emphasis added).

God is teaching me to handle others the way I do a piece of tender fruit, but also like the way I treat my own children. I am very strict and firm with my offspring. I've always been a tough disciplinarian, expecting righteous living from them, requiring that our whole family live by God's laws and principles. But when one of them sins, after the punishment or consequence, I quickly offer grace. Why? Because that's what Jesus offered. He told the woman caught in adultery that her sins were forgiven and she should "go and sin no more" (John 8:11 NLT). I bestow grace on my erring children but quickly add, "Go and sin no more."

One of my children, when confronted with a wrongdoing, told me, "Mom, it was your unexpected grace that completely blew me away." I know at the time it blew me away too. I didn't know what to say. I simply opened my mouth, probably dumbfounded, and the Holy Spirit took over, providing the perfect words!

When restoring my children, I embrace them with love and kind, thoughtful acts. And I cover their sins, never mentioning them to another soul except the Lord. (I bring everything to him over and over. He's my sounding board.) Scripture is so clear on this subject:

> Hatred stirs up strife,
> But love covers all transgressions.

Proverbs 10:12

He who covers a transgression seeks love.

Proverbs 17:9

Above all, keep fervent in your love for one another, because love covers a multitude of sins.

1 Peter 4:8

This is a difficult commandment to keep. Gossip is such a "tasty morsel" (Prov. 18:8; 26:22) and can actually be as addictive as chocolate!

Down at the nail salon . . . "Did you hear what Sally did? Yes, ran off with another man. Yes, ran off and left her dear husband and children. No, I can't believe it either. Why, I'd never do a thing like that, would you? Don't tell this to a single soul . . ."

Next customer who comes in . . . "Did you hear about Sally?" . . . Whisper, whisper, whisper!

If this had been me or my daughter who had run off, I wouldn't want a single soul to know about it. Would you? Instead, I'd want someone to cover my sin. Do I do this for others? I need to. I'm beginning to. God is teaching me to gently, kindly restore others back to fellowship. I offer them grace, God's own loving-kindness that was offered me when I least deserved it. I pursue them with prayer and good deeds. I keep their secrets, holding in my heart things I should never tell anyone but God. I ask myself often, *How would I treat my own children in this same situation? How would I want to be treated? Do unto others as I would have them do unto me . . .*

My new restoration plan is paying off big-time. We've witnessed so many prodigals return to the Lord, earthly miracles that will last through eternity. James 5:19–20 assures believers:

> "Brethren, if any among you strays from the truth and one turns him back, let him know that he who turns a sinner from the error of his way *will save his soul from death* and will cover a multitude of sins" (emphasis added).

Fruits and vegetables are for our bodies' health and sustenance in this life. But God can use them to teach us lessons that will change our lives and the lives of others forever.

4

Lean for Life

The *Healthy Balance* Way

If a genie popped out of your perfume bottle right now and promised you three wishes, what would they be? Is your number one goal to be like Christ? Would you choose that first? Would the godliness of your children be your second pick, or to win someone to Christ at work? Those are wonderful choices for a Christian woman. But what would be your third? Perhaps a little something for yourself . . . like to lose thirty pounds and become a completely new woman for your upcoming class reunion?

A recent B.C. comic strip by Johnny Hart has a cavewoman pulling the cork out of a bottle she discovered on a deserted beach. Poof! Out comes a huge genie.

"You may have one wish," he tells the woman.

Taken aback (literally, she falls on her backside!), the woman recovers and gives a firm answer: "All my life, I've wanted to be ten feet tall."

"Just out of curiosity," the genie asks, "why would a woman want to be so tall?"

"Oh, I don't really want to be tall," the woman replies dreamily. "I just wanna be *underweight!*"

Yeah, don't we all. But unless you are a female under eighteen years of age, your linear growth days are over, honey. Wishful thinking is not the way to reach your figure goals.

Guess what, though: It doesn't take a genie, a fairy godmother, or any amount of magic to lose weight. You can do that yourself—with a little support from us and a whole lot of help from the Holy Spirit. You really can do it. Others have gone before you. Just make up your mind and go for it! Atlanta pastor Charles Stanley once said, "Stamp indelibly upon your mind the person you want to become." Use fantasizing for good. Imagine how tempting you'll look lying around the pool when your husband takes you on that cruise for your tenth anniversary!

Your "New You" Notebook

Cut out the photo of that gorgeous aqua swimsuit in the catalogue, or the sleek black dress you want to wear to your reunion, or that supermodel whose shapely thighs you've always admired. Glue these inspirational pictures into your "New You" notebook, in the section entitled "Figure." Write down the changes you want to make and include the specific target dates. Make two columns labeled "Before" and "After." Take your measurements with a tape measure and record them in the first column. Measure your bustline, waistline, both arms and legs, and hips. Date the recording. Decide on a reasonable goal for changing your weight and measurements and write that down. A goal unwritten is a goal unreached. This time you really can do it!

At the top of your "Before" column, paste a total-body, scantily clad "Before" photo. (Leave room for your gorgeous

"After" photo!) Nothing motivates us like a photo, good or bad. We've destroyed various photos throughout our lifetimes. How about you? We don't want to be reminded—or have to admit—what we really look like at times! A photo reveals the truth ... bulging buns, too-tight tops, frumpy hairstyles, brown spots, and dry skin. There's no "vain imagining" that we look better than we do. That's called deception.

> Unless we change direction we are likely to end up where we are headed.
>
> ancient Chinese proverb

Repeatedly, the Bible warns Christians about deception, which is an illusion or the use of deceit. Satan uses this device to drag us into sin. Eve was deceived, and she even admitted it! In Genesis 3:13 she cries, "The serpent *deceived* me, and I ate" (emphasis added). To deceive means to make a person believe what is not true. Satan told her several half-truths: Yes, her eyes would be opened (they were), and yes, she would know good and evil (she saw she was naked and wasn't thrilled about that! "Fig tree, here I come!"). But he also told her a bold-faced lie: "You will not die." (God had said she would.) True to God's Word, in the day that Eve ate of the forbidden fruit, she began to die physically, emotionally, and spiritually.

Satan uses his little trick, deception, over and over. Christians fall for it repeatedly because they aren't aware of it. Scripture warns, "Do not be deceived . . ." (1 Cor. 3:18; 6:9; 15:33; Gal. 6:7; Eph. 5:6; 2 Thess. 2:3; 2 Tim. 3:13; James 1:16 are just a few examples).

This brings us back to our weight loss theme. If we are "carried away and enticed by our own lust" (lust for the scrumptious foods that tempt us, causing us to overindulge), how will we ever become the beautiful women of God we are longing to be?

Cynthia Shares

I didn't really understand deception until last summer. For three days, Satan severely tempted me in a way I had never experienced. I was tempted to throw in the "His and Hers" towels—I wanted to escape my difficult marriage. I didn't want to persevere any more. Satan deceived me, and of course, for those three days, I didn't break open my Bible or pray (much). I wanted to stay in my little fantasy. But then finally, thank God, I snapped myself out of it. I thought, "No, Cindy. You are not going to believe this lie. You have always followed God, and you're going to continue to obey him."

I immediately got into the Word of God. What was the truth? I needed to know! I opened right to James 1:12 (NKJV): "Blessed is the man who endures temptation; for when he has been approved, he will receive the crown of life which the Lord has promised to those who love Him."

And what was the truth? In John 15:9, 14 Jesus said, "If you keep My commandments, you will abide in My love. . . . You are My friends if you do what I command you."

I really do love Jesus Christ and want to please him. Here he tells us the way to love him: obedience to his commands. James 1:14–16 goes on to explain how we are sucked into sin: "Each one is tempted when he is carried away and enticed by his own lust. Then when lust has conceived, it gives birth to sin; and when sin is accomplished, it brings forth death. Do not be deceived, my beloved brethren."

The wages of sin is death according to Romans 6:23. Sin delivers death in so many areas of our lives: death of our relationship with God, death of godliness, death of Christian relationships, death of godly dreams. I have a godly dream of standing before Jesus Christ on that future day when he hands out rewards. The Lord will commend me for persevering in my marriage for his glory. Then he'll bring my five children up one by one and reward me for my faithfulness as a godly mother. He'll also bring forward those I've led to Christ. Crowns are nice, but these are my real jewels. This godly dream will never become a reality if I give in and give up.

This summer, I (Cynthia) persevered and did not give in to temptation. In my Bible next to a highlighted James 1:12, I penned: "July 25, 2002. Victory over temptation! All glory to God!" We have supernatural strength to do what our Lord desires of us. He will help us in our journey to perfect health in body and soul.

To Lose or Not to Lose

Obesity is a serious but common problem. Americans are deceived about it, however. When a survey was taken asking Americans how much they weighed, they always guessed below their actual weight—at least ten pounds below. Our eyes are open, but we're not seeing reality; it's only when we admit the truth about ourselves in every area, body and soul, that we will be changed. Obesity is an accepted condition in our families, our churches, our society. One in two Americans is overweight, and this year 300,000 of us will die due to weight-related illnesses. As a culture, we suffer from a two-pronged problem: *overeating* and *underexercising*. The Romans were obsessive about creating checks and balances to their physical and mental states. They would exercise more when they overate. In twenty-first-century America, we indulge in our high-fat, high-sugar, high-carb, high-calorie, low-nutrient diet while we sit in chairs at work and drive home in cushy cars to sit in our plush recliners in front of TV just before plopping into "pillow tops."

What comfort lovers we are! We pamper our posteriors and crave comfort for our stomachs (and psyches) through food. Can we become any more sedentary? Hopefully not! The most recent research reveals that the healthiest, most long-lived people weigh less than normal and eat low-calorie diets. And the ones who keep it off exercise regularly. Do you want to live a long, healthy (and attractive) life? The two-part problem has a two-part solution: *a lower-calorie, nutrient-packed diet and a high-energy exercise plan.*

How much weight do you want to lose? Don't check the Metropolitan Life Tables for Ideal Body Weight, the standard that America and its doctors go by. They've been adapted to today's high norm. Notice the chart below. Ideal body weights for women in 1959 are in parentheses, and 1983 standards are in bold type. Note the large increase in those thirty years. Imagine what it is today!

Ideal Body Weight Chart
Women

Height	Small Frame	Medium Frame	Large Frame
4'9"	**99–108** (89–95)	**106–118** (93–104)	**115–128** (101–116)
4'10"	**100–119** (91–98)	**108–120** (95–107)	**117–131** (103–119)
4'11"	**101–112** (93–101)	**110–123** (98–110)	**119–134** (106–122)
5'	**103–115** (96–104)	**112–126** (101–113)	**122–137** (109–125)
5'1"	**105–118** (99–107)	**116–129** (104–116)	**125–140** (112–128)
5'2"	**108–121** (102–110)	**118–132** (107–119)	**128–144** (115–131)
5'3"	**111–124** (105–113)	**121–135** (110–123)	**131–148** (118–135)
5'4"	**114–127** (108–116)	**124–138** (113–127)	**134–152** (122–139)
5'5"	**117–130** (111–120)	**127–141** (117–132)	**137–156** (126–143)
5'6"	**120–133** (115–124)	**130–144** (121–136)	**140–160** (130–147)
5'7"	**123–136** (119–128)	**133–147** (125–140)	**143–164** (134–151)
5'8"	**126–139** (123–132)	**136–150** (129–144)	**146–167** (138–155)
5'9"	**129–142** (127–137)	**139–153** (133–148)	**149–170** (142–160)
5'10"	**132–145** (131–141)	**142–156** (137–152)	**152–173** (146–165)
5'11"	**135–148** (135–145)	**145–159** (141–156)	**155–176** (150–170)

Recent studies suggest that adults should reduce to, or near, their high school weight, if it was normal. Was your high school weight near the 1959 standard? Didn't you feel better then? Since I've been both thick and thin, I (Cynthia) can attest that thin feels better. It feels light and energetic. It feels lean and inconspicuous. It feels good to go into a boutique, try on a dress, and have it slide easily down over my hips. Clothing choices are endless. It's so much better than having a closet full of clothes that don't fit! Being thin not only looks and feels better, it's also healthier, according to Dr. Roy Walford, author of *The 120 Year Diet.* Dr. Walford is a professor at UCLA and was the crew physician of Biosphere 2 (the glass dome that housed an experiment on diet and environmental effects on aging). Low body weight prevents many diseases, he explains, and may actually help you live longer.[1]

The Nurses' Health Study, a renowned research analysis testing 110,000 women on the effect of body weight on mortality rates, found that women with a body mass index (BMI) of 19 lived the longest.[2] And they might have been the happiest too—their clothes fit! Yes, that's skinny. No extra padding! But the huge study showed that a BMI increase from 19 to 25 increased death from all causes by 20 percent. A BMI of 28 increased mortality risk by 60 percent, and a BMI of 29 or higher increased it to over 100 percent.[3] See the chart on page 81 to figure out your BMI, which is the ratio of your body weight to your squared height.

The BMI's of top fashion models run about 18. How do they do it? How can we find our own personal lower BMI? Here again is the truth that can't be repeated too many times: The best studies show that dieters who were once obese but have maintained their new low weight for five years attribute their success to two things, *the intake of a low-fat, low-cal diet* and *the output of energy through regu-*

~~Cynthia Shares~~

The years that I followed the *Healthy Balance* plan in its strictest form, omitting most high carbs and fruit, I was very thin. But my doctor (and medical test results) kept assuring me that I was also very healthy. I had no risk of today's debilitating and deadly diseases like heart disease, high blood pressure, stroke, diabetes, and osteoporosis. It's great to have that peace of mind when you're doing all you can to stay healthy. But from a woman's point of view, lean looks and feels better, too!

---

lar physical exercise. It's simple mathematics: More calorie burning and fewer calories equals less of you.

Ideal weight standards aren't the only things that have changed in our country. The amount of food served has increased too. America's portions grow bigger by the year. Cathy Guisewite, creator of the "Cathy" comic strip, has been touching on this subject lately. One cartoon shows the standard salad, circa 1950. It's one bowl of greens. The ideal salad today is a monstrous salad bar with five hundred choices. The customary fruit serving of 1950 was one apple. Today's serving is a huge fruit platter piled high with fruit. The brown-bag lunch fifty years ago was a paper bag filled with a few food items. Today's workday lunch shows

> Everything in
> moderation.
>
> Aristotle

a refrigerator filled with Cathy's brown bags to accommodate NIH nutritional guidelines recommended for good health. It's funny . . . but it's not. Unfortunately the joke's on us, and the obese aren't laughing.

The solution comes as a change in perspective. Americans always think bigger is better, more is a must. If we want to get back to healthier (and slimmer) living, we need to

Body Mass Index Chart

	100	105	110	115	120	125	130	135	140	145	150	155	160	165	170	175	180	185	190	195	200	205
5'0"	20	21	21	22	23	24	25	26	27	28	29	30	31	32	33	34	35	36	37	38	39	40
5'1"	19	20	21	22	23	24	25	26	26	27	28	29	30	31	32	33	34	35	36	37	38	39
5'2"	18	19	20	21	22	23	24	25	26	27	27	28	29	30	31	32	33	34	35	36	37	37
5'3"	18	19	20	20	21	22	23	24	25	26	27	27	28	29	30	31	32	33	34	35	35	36
5'4"	17	18	19	20	21	21	22	23	24	25	26	27	27	28	29	30	31	32	33	33	34	35
5'5"	17	17	18	19	20	21	22	22	23	24	25	26	27	27	28	29	30	31	32	33	33	34
5'6"	16	17	18	19	19	20	21	22	23	23	24	25	26	27	27	28	29	30	31	31	32	33
5'7"	16	16	17	18	19	20	20	21	22	23	23	24	25	26	27	27	28	29	30	31	31	32
5'8"	15	16	17	17	18	19	20	21	21	22	23	24	24	25	26	27	27	28	29	30	30	31
5'9"	15	16	16	17	18	18	19	20	21	21	22	23	24	24	25	26	27	27	28	29	30	30
5'10"	14	15	16	17	17	18	19	19	20	21	22	22	23	24	25	25	26	27	27	28	29	29
5'11"	14	15	15	16	17	17	18	19	20	20	21	22	22	23	24	24	25	26	26	27	28	29
6'0"	14	14	15	16	16	17	18	18	19	20	20	21	22	22	23	24	24	25	26	26	27	28
6'1"	13	14	15	15	16	16	17	18	18	19	20	20	21	22	22	23	24	24	25	26	26	27
6'2"	13	13	14	15	15	16	17	17	18	19	19	20	21	21	22	23	23	24	24	25	26	26
6'3"	12	13	14	14	15	16	16	17	17	18	19	19	20	21	21	22	22	23	24	24	25	26
6'4"	12	13	13	14	15	15	16	16	17	18	18	19	19	20	21	21	22	23	23	24	24	25

Cynthia Shares

Maintaining my normal weight grows more difficult as I approach fifty. I'd love to blame it on a "mid-life hormone crisis," but God won't let me do that. He doesn't want me to deceive myself and wants me to know the truth so I can be free. The problem is that I gave up moderation long ago. I eat far more than I ever should, worshiping the taste of food instead of being truly grateful for the fuel. I use food as entertainment. I feed my emotional needs instead of my body's health needs. I give priority to my tastebuds when I should be a good steward of the health and fit body God gave me.

I've thought about why obesity isn't acceptable in our culture. Is it simply because our society emphasizes the Body Beautiful? As I've struggled with this problem myself—gaining weight, not fitting into my clothes, yet giving in to even more temptations, overindulging more often than not, and then not wanting people to see me or not wanting to attend special events when I'm at my "high" weight—I realize that the unacceptability is shame-based. We know it's not what God had planned for our bodies. That's why we must recognize that gluttony is a sin if we are ever to be free from it. The drunk knows shame when he's discovered unconscious on the doorstep. The adulteress knows shame when she's "caught in the act." We overeaters know shame when our "lusts of the flesh" show up on our hips, thighs, and tummies.

Feel hopeless? We're not offering you some new diet plan that "just might work this time." We have something—Someone—so much greater. The Holy Spirit was sent to give us the power to be all that God plans us to be. He works *every time* we say yes to him! It feels so good to obey God's laws—yes, even his law of moderation. Check out Romans 7:18–25. The apostle Paul had some of these same struggles, but he knew where to find victory.

Use the *Healthy Balance* nutrition and exercise plan, but bring the promised Helper along as your personal trainer. Ask for his strength every day, every hour, as often as you need to. The Holy Spirit, along with your commitment and effort, can transform you into all you could ever hope to be.

change our thinking to a more biblical pattern. Moderation in all things is the Bible's motto we must adopt. That's why the second secret in our *Healthy Balance* plan is: *Practice moderation in all things.*

The *Healthy Balance* Plan for Weight Loss

In chapter 3 we shared the *Healthy Balance* nutrition program. Now we'll tell you how you can apply it to your daily life to lose weight quickly and healthfully.

Your shelves, frig, and freezer are stocked with *Healthy Balance* foods. You've experimented with several of the recipes in chapter 5. Your Balanced Butter is ready and so is a big pitcher of green tea. You've created a delicious, nutritious soup and a tempting salad, and hopefully a pot of tasty beans. And you feel quite domestic about the whole thing—healthy eating can make you feel downright smug! Just enjoy it. Before long, casual observers will be asking how you've lost so much weight and where you get all your energy.

With pen and paper, plan the week's meals. The way we ensure the perfect quantity of fresh vegetables and fruits in our diets is through soups, salads, and fresh juices. You can incorporate these into your program too.

Then organize your meals. We want to fit those daily 10 servings of fruits and vegetables into the plan. And you need low-fat protein, 1 to 2 servings of nonfat dairy, several grain and/or legume portions, and some healthy fats for nutrition and flavor.

Be creative when you plan your meals. Here are some guidelines to help you. Each day's menu should include:

Protein—3 servings: lean meats, poultry, fish, eggs, soy, combinations like beans and corn or brown rice. One serving is 3 oz of beef, poultry, pork, or fish (about the size of a deck of cards); 2 whole eggs (or 1 whole egg and 2 egg whites); or ½–1 cup of cooked legumes eaten with ½–1 cup cooked whole grain forms a complete protein.

Dairy—1 or 2 servings: 1 cup of fat-free milk, yogurt, cottage cheese, 1–2 ounces of low-fat cheese, or buttermilk. (We always have 1 cup of live-culture nonfat yogurt daily, and often an extra cup of skim milk.) Does milk really do a body good? To drink or not to drink? That is the burning question. A study published in the January 2003 American Society for Nutritional Sciences's *Journal of Nutrition* proved that women who consumed milk, yogurt, and cheese several times a day lost 70 percent more weight and 64 percent more body fat than women who didn't.[4] Components in the milk, including calcium, supercharge the metabolism to burn more fat. Substitutes in the study like broccoli, calcium-fortified orange juice, and supplements didn't work. Besides, nothing tastes quite as good with a spicy bowl of chili as the white stuff, right?

High-carbohydrates—four servings of carbs like brown rice, whole-wheat bread, corn tortillas, legumes; or high-carbohydrate vegetables are potatoes (white and sweet), yams, corn, peas, beans, pumpkin, and winter squash. A serving is 1 slice, 1 cup cold cereal, or ½ cup hot cereal, rice, or pasta, 1 small potato, or ½ cup serving.

Fats—2 Tbs a day for health and flavoring. Choose good fats like olive oil, canola and flaxseed oil, and nuts or nut oils. Avocados also provide good fat. You can also use a small amount of low-fat mayo and butter. What matters is the accumulation over the week. If one day is short on fats, you can make it up the next day. If you eat too many fats one day . . . oops, accidents do happen! Then cut back on them the next day. Fats should only total 20–25 percent of your calories. Check labels and buy foods with 20 percent fat or lower. Or see a fat gram counter. (We use fat-free sprays for cooking, good fats for flavoring—Balanced Butter on brown rice, low-fat mayo on a softened corn tortilla, garlic dressing on crisp greens. Mmmm!)

Fruits—2 or 3 servings. A serving is ½ cup cut-up fruit, or 1 piece, or 6 oz of juice. (We vary on this. Charity loves fruit. Cynthia couldn't eat fruit for many years, but now she enjoys fruit nearly every day. Usually she loads up on vegetables, though.)

Vegetables—7 or 8 servings. One serving is ½ cup cooked or raw, 1 cup leafy, or 6 oz juice. Salads, soups, and juices can provide several veggie servings in one dish. Always have 2 or 3 veggies accompanying your entrees at lunch and dinner. We even fix them at breakfast on occasion. Toss chopped onions, bell pepper, tomatoes, and mushrooms into low-fat omelettes. Spoon spicy salsa over scrambled eggs. Bake some low fat carrot muffins or warm up a prebaked yam or sweet potato. Enjoy a glass of fresh-squeezed carrot juice. You can eat low-carb veggies all day long if you want! When you get hungry, cook a vegetable or grab some carrot sticks to crunch on. (Cynthia sneaks veggies into everything! Check out some of her recipes in chapter 5. See how you can fit more vegetables into your life and let us know.)

A "Reality" *Healthy Balance* Example

Reality shows are all the rage right now. I (Cynthia) thought it might help you to see how I make the *Healthy Balance* plan work in my own life. I like to eat my protein, dairy, and produce during the day. I often save my high-carbs for a reward meal in the evening. That's when I crave comfort foods! You might like to do the same thing. For instance, at breakfast and lunch choose protein foods like lean meats, poultry, and fish, eggs or soy. Eat lots of veggies and your soups and salads at these meals too. Snacks can be fruit and yogurt. Then at dinner feast on a baked potato topped with chili, onions, and nonfat sour cream or low-fat shredded cheese. Whole-grain pasta and vegetarian sauce is another possibility, or try baked yams or squash with fruit as dessert. When I'm in a reducing mode, because I am fairly active, I eat 1350–1450 calories. Breakfasts are around 300 calories; lunches tally in at approximately 350 calories; and dinners add up to 450 or so. Snacks fill in the calorie counts.

In my "New You" notebook, I keep a journal of the foods I eat and their calories. But most important, I keep track of the fruits and vegetables I consume daily. The goal is 10 servings a day. When I exceed that number, I'm really happy with myself! To keep my metabolic rate from dropping to a slow crawl while dieting, I exercise twice a day, in the morning and evening. I also pray during this time, so it's very productive. Good for both body and soul. (We women are multitaskers!) I record my exercise for the day in my notebook too, and my prayer requests and dated answers.

Sometimes if I'm not hungry in the evening or I've eaten too much during the day, I'll forego dinner and eat some fruit or drink a glass of skim milk. That usually gives me even greater weight loss in the morning! I'll share several actual menus from this week (complete with stupid choices!). It may seem like I occasionally repeat the same foods, because I tend to do that. If something tastes really good, I want it the next day. And maybe the next . . . until I get tired of it. If you wonder about the exercise sessions spread throughout each day, that isn't always normal. When I'm sitting at a desk a lot working on some writing that's due, I break up the day with exercise. My normal routine is to do my circuit session in the morning (see page 195) and Prayer-walk in the evening.

Here is how my week balanced out:

Monday

Breakfast

Coffee with cream: 200 calories! (Unnecessary . . . use nonfat creamer.)

Soy shake made with frozen banana and skim milk: 300 calories (Very filling, no need for a snack before lunch)

(Thought process: *500 calories for breakfast—yikes! I'm going to have to adjust other meals.*)

Lunch

½ salmon filet (3 oz) baked with fresh mushrooms, onions, and garlic

Green salad with fresh lemon and 1 tsp flax oil

Asparagus steamed with lemon

275 calories for lunch

Snack
Fresh vegetable juice (three carrots/1 celery/kale/cuke):
135 calories

Whole-grain toast with ½ avocado: 295 calories

Dinner
Vegetable soup, 1 cup: 100 calories

Fresh pineapple (five slices): 100 calories

Cauliflower (½ cup): 12 calories

Baked winter squash: 70 calories

Day's total input: 1487 calories

Fruit: 3

Vegetables: 20

Total: 23! Hooray for me!

Day's output (exercise): A.M. half-hour jog; Noon half-hour circuit weight training; P.M. half-hour jog/walk

Tuesday

Breakfast
Coffee with creamer: 40 calories

Whole-grain toast and other half of avocado: 295 calories

Lunch
Other half salmon filet with mushrooms, onions, garlic: 185 calories

Homemade vegetable soup: 100 calories

Salad with 1 Tbs flax oil and apple cider vinegar: 125 calories

Snack
Fresh vegetable juice: 70 calories

Dinner

Soy shake with skim milk and frozen bananas: 340 calories

Snack

Roasted almonds (¼ cup): 170 calories

Skim milk, 1 cup: 100 calories

Day's total input: 1425 calories

Fruit: 2

Veggies: 12

Total: 14

Day's output: A.M. half-hour jog/walk; P.M. twenty minutes minitramp, twenty minutes stretching

Wednesday

Breakfast

Coffee with creamer: 40 calories

Juice of 1 lemon in water

Vegi-egg omelette (1 whole egg, 2 whites, veggies): 240 calories

Sauteed veggies like mushrooms, onions, bell pepper folded into the omelette

Lunch

Vegetable soup, 1 cup: 100 calories

Plain, fat-free yogurt, 1 cup: 200 calories

Dinner

Friends called us to go out to dinner—saved up calories for this!

Ricardo's Tostada with Garlic Dressing and Salsa: 750 calories

> Veggies and salsa (slices of jicama, zucchini, bell pepper, and celery brought from home for dipping—the chips are diet destroyers!): 50 calories
>
> Iced tea

Day's total input: 1380 calories

Fruit: 1

Veggies: 13

Total: 14

Day's output: A.M. half-hour jog/walk; Noon half-hour circuit weight training

That's enough of an example to give you an idea of a plan that works for me. In those three days I lost three pounds! The week was atypical though, as Monday morning a storm caused an electrical outage. I was unable to make my usual homemade soup and a pot of beans. We were forced to eat leftovers, but when they are good and healthy too, who cares?

Don't forget: Calories count. Not only the ones you take in, but the ones you use up. As you follow the *Healthy Balance* nutrition plan, remember to add some physical activity every day.

A Sample Menu Plan for the Week

Have fun experimenting with these meals from the recipe section. Here's a one-week sample menu plan:

Monday—Day One

1390 calories

Fruit: 3
Vegetables: 15
Total: 18!

Breakfast: 300 calories

Juice of 1 lemon in cup of water while cooking breakfast.

Tricolor Omelette (1 yolk, 2 whites) with three veggies: chopped onions, bell peppers, tomatoes, or mushrooms (see recipe page 124)

Coffee (can use creamer, nonfat canned milk; cream must be counted as fat)

Snack: 100 calories

Large orange

Lunch: 280 calories

Cup of Vegetable Soup (see recipe page 115)

2 cups salad with 1 Tbs olive oil and basalmic vinegar, ½ cup cooked kidney beans and ¼ cup tiny cooked shrimp added

Iced green tea (may use artificial sweetener)

Snack: 300 calories

Banana, cup of fat-free yogurt, plain or sweetened with aspartame

Dinner: 410 calories

Crunchy Coleslaw, ½ cup (see recipe page 125)

Chicken-and-Cheese Calzones (see recipe page 127)

1 cup broccoli with lemon

Hot tea

Tuesday—Day Two

1435 calories
Fruit: 3

Vegetables: 11
Total: 14

Breakfast: 280 calories
Juice of 1 lime in 1 cup of water
Traditional oatmeal, 1 cup (see recipe page 124)
1 cup fat-free or 1 percent milk for cereal and drinking
1 fresh peach
Coffee or hot tea

Snack: 80 calories
Medium apple

Lunch: 450 calories
Open-faced turkey sandwich: 1 slice whole-wheat bread, mustard, 2 oz of turkey breast, slices of lettuce (or sprouts), tomato, and red onion
1 cup beans

Snack: 200 calories
Yogurt, nonfat blueberry, 1 cup

Dinner: 425 calories
Tomato, three slices, with 1 tsp low-fat mayo, and 1 cup salad
Roasted Garlic Chicken, 3 oz (see recipe page 128)
½ cup carrots, small onion, roasted with chicken
Small roasted potato

Wednesday—Day Three

1420 calories
Fruit: 4
Vegetables: 9
Total: 13

Breakfast: 300 calories
  Juice of 1 lime in 1 cup of water
  Breakfast Shake: fruit smoothie (see recipe page 124)
  or soy breakfast shake from mix

Snack with a friend: 100 calories
  Coffee with 1 Tbs half-and-half, plain biscotti

Lunch: 400 calories
  Vegetable soup
  ½ avocado filled with tuna salad: made with chopped
    celery and 2 tsp low-fat mayo; small garden salad on
    the side with lemon
  Iced green tea

Snack: 200 calories
  Plain, fat-free yogurt or light yogurt

Dinner: 420 calories
  Vegetable soup, 1 cup
  2 cups salad with 1 Tbs olive or flax oil and balsamic
    vinegar
  Colorful Crustless Quiche (see recipe page 129)

Snack:
  Hot fruit-flavored tea (may use artificial sweetener)

Thursday—Day Four

1420 calories
Fruit: 3
Vegetables: 7
Total: 10

Breakfast: 330 calories
  Lemon juice in cup of water
  Whole-grain toast with 1 Tbs peanut butter

2 kiwi

Coffee with creamer

Snack: 200 calories

Plain yogurt, or light, 1 cup

Lunch: 330 calories

Baked corn tortilla, ½ cup fat-free refried beans

2 cups salad with 1 oz low-fat cheddar, shredded on
top

½ cup salsa poured over top of tostada

Diet soda

Snack: 60 calories

Fresh cantaloupe (¼ melon)

Dinner: 500 calories

Vegetable soup, ½ cup

Green salad with 1 Tbs Italian dressing (see recipe page
126)

Meatless Italian sauce (see recipe page 131) over ¾ cup
whole-grain pasta

Cracked wheat roll with 1 tsp Balanced Butter

Friday—Day Five

1360 calories

Fruit: 3

Vegetables: 8

Total: 11

Breakfast: 350 calories

Juice of 1 lemon in water

Slice of toasted whole-grain bread with 1 Tbs almond
butter

1 slice (2 inch) of watermelon

Coffee with creamer

Snack: 65 calories

Whole orange

Lunch: 390 calories

Balance Beans with Chili, 1 cup (see recipe pages 121)

Corn Bread (see recipe page 126), 1 tsp Balanced Butter

1 cup skim milk

Snack: 200 calories

Plain fat-free yogurt, 1 cup

Dinner: 355 calories

Restaurant:

Salad (1 cup) with 1 Tbs oil and vinegar

Grilled salmon with lemon

Broccoli or vegetable side

Coffee with creamer (you can bring nonfat creamer from home, and if you start your hot drink before dinner, you'll fill up faster)

Saturday—Day Six

1450 calories

Fruit: 4

Vegetables: 10

Total: 14

Breakfast: 370 calories

Juice of 1 lime in water

1 cup dry cereal: Shredded Wheat, Raisin Bran, or Grape-nuts, with 1 banana

½ cup skim milk for cereal

Coffee with creamer

Snack: 80 calories

Fresh vegetable juice or piece of fruit

Lunch: 280 calories

Bowl vegetable soup

Baked Vegetables or Charity's Italian Vegi-Bake (see recipes pages 127 and 130)

Snack: 200 calories

Cup of plain, unsweetened yogurt or light

Dinner: 450 calories

Marinated Steak (3–4 oz), barbecued (see recipe page 129)

Skinny Mashed Potatoes, 1 cup (see recipe page 127)

Salad, 1 cup, with 1 Tbs Marie's Blue Cheese dressing

Sliced steamed zucchini, ½ cup

Dessert: 70 calories

Charity's Raspberry Refresher (see recipe page 131)

Sunday—Day Seven

1395 calories

Fruit: 2

Vegetables: 8

Total: 10

Sunday Brunch: 630 calories

Reward Meal! Enjoy!

Orange juice, 6 oz

2 whole-grain waffles with low-cal syrup (¼ cup) or sugar-free fruit jam (3 tsp)

1 egg, scrambled in 1 tsp butter

3 slices crisp bacon

2 cups coffee with 2 Tbs half-n-half

Afternoon snack: 180 calories

Light microwave popcorn, 1 bag, or ⅛ cup almonds

Fresh Vegetable Juice (see recipe page 125)

Iced diet soda or tea

Dinner: 460 calories

1 cup salad with 1 Tbs oil and vinegar

Vegi-Grain Saute (see recipe page 129)

Dessert: 125 calories

Pronto Pudding Parfaits (see recipe page 132)

Substitute: Fat-free Heavenly Dessert (add 35 calories to day's total; see recipe page 132)

These sample meals give you an idea how you can create a *Healthy Balance* menu for a week. There are options for hurried days, for lazy days, for brown-bag days, and for special days. Each day's menu satisfies your quota of vegetables and fruit. Although vitamin packed, these menus add up to only 1350–1450 calories a day! (You never want to go lower than 1200 calories a day. Below that, your metabolism slows and burns fewer calories. If you exercise a lot, keep your day's total around 1400.) In addition, the *Healthy Balance* plan spreads your calories throughout the day. This boosts your metabolism every time you eat. You'll lose weight fast but stay healthy, strong, and satisfied.

Adaptations for the *Healthy Balance* Diet

The *Healthy Balance* plan is a great way to eat whether you have pounds to lose or not. We compiled the program after years of research, emphasizing what the body truly needs for good nutrition. But you can also adapt the program to your individual needs and your current lifestyle.

Faster Weight Loss

If you have pounds to shed and want to lose them sooner rather than later, cut out your high-carbs and fruit for several weeks. The pounds melt away! Foods that are high in carbohydrates include white potatoes, white flour and its products, honey and sugar and products made with them, white rice, grains, dairy, and legumes. Instead, eat protein foods like lean meats, poultry, fish, egg whites and soy; low-carb vegetables like leafy green salads, green vegetables, cruciferous vegetables like cabbage and broccoli, celery, cucumbers, garlic, onions (not sweet), mushrooms, bell peppers, summer squash, and zucchini. Add some healthy oils and even some sugar-free salad dressings for flavor. Fat isn't the issue here as much as high-glycemic foods, which create a surge in insulin when you eat them. This extra insulin is stored as fat, in addition to putting a strain on your body. During this quick weight loss phase of the *Healthy Balance* diet, keep your carbohydrates at 20 grams a day or less. (Purchase a carbohydrate or glycemic gram counter.) After several weeks of this low-carb discipline, begin to add the other foods on the list (see page 79) one or two at a time. Watch the scale to be sure you keep losing. Try to keep your calorie count for each day between 1300 and 1400. Also, eat some protein at each meal. These two strategies (plus the addition of daily exercise) will continue the weight loss without lowering your metabolism.

Use these guidelines to figure out how many calories you need:

To maintain weight: multiply your present weight by

    12, if you are inactive

    15, if moderately active

    20, if extremely active

To reduce: subtract 500 calories a day from normal diet to lose 1 pound a week through diet alone. Exercise will increase this loss.

Expectant mothers: add 300 nonfat calories daily to prepregnancy count

Lactating mothers: add 500 nonfat calories to prepregnancy count

For Vegetarians

Many people are trying to limit or eliminate the animal foods they ingest. Research has demonstrated that a plant-based diet can produce excellent health, and studies have shown that we were originally created to consume plant foods. Carnivores have the extra length in their intestines necessary for the prolonged assimilation of animal proteins. Humans, on the other hand, have shorter G.I. tracts perfect for digesting fruits, vegetables, grains, legumes, and seeds. But some people just seem to need a heavier diet that includes meat.

Should you eat meat? That will be up to you to decide. Since God did offer it to humankind (after the flood, and then again in the New Testament vision to the apostle Peter), we see no religious reason not to include meat, poultry, and fish in the *Healthy Balance* plan for weight loss. What would Jesus do? Well, we know for sure that he ate fish on occasion. We have tried to include in our plan all the best God has offered to us. (However, in our next LifeBalance series book, *The Inner Balance,* we offer a completely plant-based diet, free of all animal products, to use in a cleansing program.) Generally, we try to limit the amount of animal protein (including fish) we eat to two to three times a week (when we are not on a weight loss diet and can consume plenty of carbohydrates).

If you are vegetarian, however, you can still enjoy the *Healthy Balance* plan. Actually, you'll go crazy over the quantity of vegetables and fruits offered on this program! Include more complex carbohydrates like brown rice, corn, rye, oats, and legumes. Eat grains and legumes together at several daily meals. They combine to provide complete protein. Instead of the Balanced Butter, you can purchase a soy substitute spread like Soy Garden, available at some supermarkets and most health food stores. Also available are soy cheeses and beverages. Nuts make a tasty meat substitute for all of us. And unlike animal fat, the fats that nuts contribute to our bodies are healthy oils, like monounsaturated and polyunsaturated oils (these will help your body utilize insulin and lower cholesterol, among other advantages). A study done at the Harvard School of Public Health revealed that nut munchers gain no more weight than those who don't regularly consume nuts. Use self-control, however. Roasted, salted almonds are like the old potato chip ad: "Bet you can't eat just one!" One-fourth cup of almonds equals 170 calories, most of those from good fats. Portion control your nuts or eat them with a meal so you don't overdo them.

Pregnancy and Lactation

The *Healthy Balance* plan is a wonderful plan while eating for two. You will receive all the nourishment that your body and your baby need at this time. Check with your physician. My obstetrician encouraged me (Cynthia) to stay on this eating program while I was pregnant. The pregnancies when I ate this way went wonderfully: I felt super, didn't gain unnecessary weight, and lost the extra "baby baggage" the first month after delivery. And my babies were so healthy! When I didn't stick with this plan while pregnant, I ran into some serious problems with both health and weight. We suggest that you up your calorie count to at least 1500 calories a day during this time, though. And while lactating, you can add even more servings of each food category. Milk production uses many calories. Add the extra calories into your snack times. That way you aren't overeating at meals, which can put a strain on your body and prompt fat storage.

The Patriotic Snack Attack

Snacking. It's an all-American pastime. The snack attack may account for some of our country's obesity. We realize that everyone occasionally gets hit by a snack attack, though, so we have to be realistic and give you some ideas to try when the mood strikes.

Craving a flavored cold beverage? You can have a diet soda occasionally, but avoid them on a daily basis. Choose iced tea (sweetened with a packet of artificial sweetener or the herbal stevia, if desired). Iced tea is my beverage of choice anytime (Charity). It always has been. Black and green teas are loaded with antioxidants and cathechins to protect DNA, to guard against disease, and to retard aging. I brew 2 gallons of flavored herbal tea at the beginning of each week. Personal favorites are mint and citrus green tea. While the hot tea is cooling, I add sweetener or honey. It dissolves more thoroughly while the tea is warm. Then I pour it into a 2-gallon glass jug and keep it cool and ready in the fridge. Cynthia's sister, Sandy, favors equal parts tea and prepared flavored Crystal Light (sweetened with aspartame). If artificial sweeteners are no problem for you, make a pitcher of this mix, pour some into a tall glass of ice, and enjoy.

When you have a carb craving, the best cure is butter-flavored, reduced-fat microwave popcorn. You can eat the whole bag and not upset your diet! (You count it as 2 carb servings, plus you'll be getting lots of necessary fiber.) The popcorn, along with your diet soda or flavored tea, should satisfy you until dinner. Or try some carrot and celery sticks (precut and bagged at the store) dipped into low-fat Ranch dressing. Author Mark Twain sat around crunching cauliflower while he composed his best-sellers. He was convinced that the vegetable contributed to his creativity. I (Cynthia) have tried it—you can tell me if it works!

Want something sweet instead? Sugar-free, fat-free hot cocoa or pudding indulges a sugar and chocolate longing at the same time. Have a desire to splurge on dessert? Fix some sugar-free Jell-O (your favorite flavor). After it has set, mix in some fat-free whipped cream and even some chopped fruit. Stick it into the freezer. Once frozen, you can enjoy it like you would ice cream.

We hate diet programs that assume you'll never fight the urge to cheat. Here are several things to sneak in when you can no longer control yourself (don't worry, they won't sabotage all your efforts!):

1 cup fat-free, sugar-free pudding in favorite flavor

1 scoop fat-free, sugar-free ice cream in favorite flavor

1 frozen all-juice bar

45 pretzel sticks

1 biscotti with coffee

Whole-grain toast with 1 Tbs fruit butter or preserves

Some healthy seeds or nuts (full of good fats) but not
    too many

You can have hot tea or coffee with any of these treats. And remember, if you actually get hungry any time during the day or night, have more of your soup or salad! Also try drinking water. In America our craving mechanisms are out of whack. Sometimes we feel like we just want "something," and we don't know what it is. We forage around in the kitchen (the old hunter-gatherer coming out in us!) when what we really want is a drink of pure, refreshing water. When you get a craving, try drinking a big glass of H_2O first. Wait a few minutes and see if your "hungries" calm down because it was really thirst that was calling. Experts say that any craving will go away if you wait fifteen minutes before indulging it. Go indulge in a distraction instead!

The day may come, however, when you "fall off the wagon," dietwise. Don't give up. That's the worst thing that can happen. We've seen women who are doing so well losing weight and gaining a huge portion of self-esteem. Something happens. The holidays arrive and so do all those tantalizing goodies, too good to resist. They eat one, two, maybe three at the most. But that does it. They've blown it and believe they can't be redeemed. Feeling overblown guilt, they give up and go crazy on junk food. They gain back the weight and often a pound or two extra—so discouraging. Don't let yourself fall into that trap physically, psychologically, and spiritually. Satan has set the trap for you—avoid the snares of the devil!

The Devil Made Me Do It

Falling off the wagon. That happens to many Christians who are trying so hard to live for God. They go along in life, obedient and doing so well. A crisis or temptation comes, or perhaps a harsh criticism. They feel bad and walk away from God. Or maybe they just ignore him for a while. They choose to sin. Then, instead of getting right back on the spiritual "wagon," they are so discouraged with themselves that they keep stumbling along behind. More sin, more regret, more shame. Finally, they fall flat on their faces. They give up and choose the wide, easy path where sinners walk. They are just where Satan wants them!

Don't let the enemy sabotage your diet, your growth, your goals and dreams. When you make bad choices, whether in your diet or in your life, simply seek God's forgiveness. Pick yourself up and follow the path that you've chosen, the one you know is right, the path that leads to a better life—to eternal life.

Those of us pursuing health and fitness for body and soul have chosen the road less traveled. We came to a fork in the road, whether spiritually when our sins caught up with us and the Truth was revealed, or physically when we were finally too sick to get out of bed or too chubby to zip our pants. We chose the narrow way, and now we're going against our culture. The world says, "Don't believe the Bible. There are many ways to heaven; Jesus isn't the only way. You really don't have to take Scripture literally. You don't have to obey those commandments. You'll get into heaven by being the good person you are. You don't need to read the Bible and pray. You don't need the Holy Spirit; you can handle this church work on your own." On and on the deceptive brainwashing goes. The world encourages us, "Eat, drink, and be merry. Tomorrow you're going to die anyway, so indulge in your passions. Don't deny yourself. Live it up. There really aren't any consequences."

The way that the world travels is broad, easy, and packed with people. You've chosen the narrow way. Jesus said that few ever find it. Take heart! You are on the right path. Just keep following him, and you'll get to the Promised Land!

On the *Healthy Balance* diet, if you blow it one day (or in an evening out to dinner), just cut back the next. Weight loss results from the total calories taken in and used up throughout the week (input and output). If you blow it too many days in a row, you'll show a weight gain, naturally (ask us, we know!). But one "I fell off the wagon" day won't destroy your diet, so don't let it.

Sometimes we just need a little help from a friend. The following are some sly strategies that will almost make you forget you're dieting. They work for us!

A Dieter's Tricks

Use a smaller plate. America's dinner plate has grown over the past twenty years from ten inches to fourteen, and it's still growing. I (Cynthia) will never forget our first dinner out with our dear friends John and Barbara Palermo. When Barbara's plate and mine arrived, they were the biggest at the table, huge platters of food. We all laughed. I jokingly commented, "You are a girl after my own heart, Barbara." We were instant cohorts in cuisinary crime from that moment on! Your low-cal foods will look lost on a large platter. Instead, choose a luncheon or salad plate and fill it with just the right amount of food (up to 2 cups—½ cup protein, ½ cup starch, 1 cup veggies) to stay fit!

Drink water before a meal. A cup of hot tea or coffee works even better to fill your stomach with something before the food hits. Research has shown that soup eaters who begin their meal with a hot bowl of broth lose the most weight. Continue to drink pure water throughout the day. You need 8–10 cups to rehydrate. Don't trust your thirst mechanism. Train yourself to drink the water your body needs.

Eat dessert first. Bet you determined to obey this suggestion the minute you read it, right? Just kidding, unfortunately. But do eat some fat. Fats give you a satisfied feeling faster than other foods. If you eat them early in the meal, you'll consume fewer calories overall. Begin your meal with salad topped with dressing or vinegar and oil. Or try some crudités (cut-up veggies) with low-fat ranch dressing. A vegetable side dish topped with 1 tsp of rich, creamy butter. A small handful of nuts. A scoop of guacamole with baked cornmeal chips—ole!

Don't tempt yourself. Plan meals based on the same healthy foods while using a variety of fruits and vegetables to add excitement to your diet. A study at Tufts University proved that a variety of food in any category except fruits and vegetables caused subjects to overeat and become obese. Increasing the variety of fruits had no effect on body weight. But increasing the variety of vegetables caused even greater weight loss! More praise for green things!

Feed on demand. That's a breast-feeding term. Lots of mothers swear by it. It can work for dieters too. Eat when you're hungry and not when the clock (or someone else) tells you to. Wait until you hear that familiar growl. Or maybe it's not too familiar to you. Reacquaint yourself with true hunger (but not a famished feeling). Feel that rumble in your stomach. Then eat. You'll enjoy your food more—and eat less. Snacking piles on the pounds.

Know when to stop. There's the catch. It's not too hard for us to be sure when we're hungry. It's much more difficult to tell when we're satisfied. Most of us lost our appetite control mechanism after childhood. Watch children. Pile food on their plates. It doesn't matter how scrumptious it is, when kids are finished, they're finished. They can't be talked into another bite. "No, I'm full," comes a firm answer. If they are ever coerced into overeating, they shove their plates back, make a face, rub their tummies, and groan, "Ugh! I'm full. My stomach hurts."

Eat more to burn more. This trick sounds like it contradicts the last one. But every time you eat something, your metabolism kicks in to burn the calories. So don't stuff yourself once, twice, three times a day. Research shows that people who eat most of their calories at one sitting gain the most weight (like those who skip breakfast and lunch and indulge themselves at dinner). Keep that light feeling in mind. Spread your food allotment throughout the day. Since you're eating mostly fruits and vegetables, you won't be loading up on fats and high-carbs. But you will be revving up your calorie-burning metabolism.

Reward yourself. Many dieters punish themselves when they fall off the low-cal wagon. Don't! Commit yourself to a lifetime of healthful eating and climb back on! (After all, don't you want to look and feel good for the rest of your long life, and not just for that reunion?) Once you are at normal weight, eat healthy all week, and then present yourself with a reward meal on the weekend (perhaps at your favorite restaurant). Or buy yourself a gift if you stay on your eating plan for the next three weeks. How about that aqua swimsuit? Or better yet, talk your husband into buying it for you. It's kind of like a gift for him too, right? Treat yourself to a movie at the end of a good week. Whatever it takes, but just don't punish yourself. That becomes a vicious cycle in which you'll eat to feel comforted.

Yo-yos are no-nos. Crash dieting damages the body, disrupting DNA and lowering metabolism. Aim for health. Don't go for the fads. You may lose a lot of weight fast but end up in bed, unable to show off your new figure!

Try a taste. Sometimes all you really need is a tiny taste of something delicious. You don't really need to eat the whole thing! Instead of a bowl of ice cream, scoop one spoonful out of the container and savor that. You can't dip the spoon back in, so throw it in the sink. Out to dinner? Don't order dessert. Eat one bite of your husband's treat. End the meal with a sweet taste. Some dentists say not to chew gum, as it stresses the jaw joint. But I (Cynthia) chew peppermint gum a lot. It's the minty taste I'm craving, so I'll pop in a piece after a meal. It keeps my mouth busy and out of trouble! (Plus I'm not crazy about bad breath.) Or try brushing your teeth with fresh-smelling toothpaste. It leaves a sweet, clean taste in your mouth that you'll learn to love.

Keep a food diary. In your "New You" notebook, write down the foods you eat each day and the circumstances surrounding the meal, snack, or food attack (i.e. binge). Many studies have shown that dieters who keep a food journal lose the most weight. Notice any patterns. Do you always grab a chocolate bar after a stressful call from your mom? Are you an afternoon binger? Or do you get yearnings at night in front of the TV? Note the food items you are eating. With your goal of health in mind, are they nutritious?

Cynthia Shares

I always laugh at my kids when we go out to dinner and they "pig out." All the way home, I hear complaints from the backseat. "Adults get used to pigging out and feeling miserable," I joke with them. "You have to train yourself to eat past the point of pain." More groans from the backseat of the car.

Of course, I'm just kidding them. But isn't it the truth? As kids, we didn't gorge. At some point as we grew older, we learned to love the taste of food more than we loved the light feel of our bodies after a moderate meal.

Aim for that light, satisfied feeling after every meal rather than that "overeater's ache." It can become as addictive as overeating. It's all in your eating habits.

Be sure you are getting your 10 fruits and veggies a day and your 8 cups of water.

Develop diversions. If a craving calls, call a friend. Chat for about fifteen minutes, the time it takes for the hankering to become history. Other distractions that work fine: a sport, a pet, an entertaining novel or TV program (except perhaps a cooking show!). When the craving strikes, jump on your trampoline for fifteen minutes or take a walk. That way you're working the old "kill two birds with one stone" motto!

Exchange cardio for carbs. Dopamine and serotonin are two chemicals in the brain that are pleasure producing. They are released when we overeat. A binge on carbohydrates— candy, cookies, cake, chocolate, potato chips, fries—floods our brains and bodies with feelings of satisfaction, calm, comfort, and pleasure. That's why food has such a soothing effect. No wonder we eat those things—that's a lot of bang for our buck! Drugs like Prozac are much more expensive! Aerobic exercise does the same thing, releasing the "feel-good hormones" with no weight gain. When down in the dumps, talk yourself into a five-minute walk. Once you're out there, the fresh air and physical movement will lift your spirits, encouraging you to continue on.

Seek support. Studies reveal that dieters who feel supported by family and friends lose the most weight and keep it off. Join a weight watchers group of some sort, or create one. Recruit a friend. Try on-line support groups. Another aspect of involving others in your diet plan can be broadcasting to several key people that you're going to lose X amount of pounds by X date. It will motivate you to shoot for that goal and hit it. Embarrassment is a great motivator!

Speed up. One of my (Charity's) biggest weapons against overeating is staying busy. It's when I'm bored and lazy that I think constantly about eating to entertain myself. I just can't allow myself time to sit and snack. When I'm mentally focused on a task, I become completely unaware of my growling stomach and can actually go without eating for hours at a time. Not allowing my mind to dwell on my cravings is key. Clean the garage. Go shopping. Run errands. Window-shop with a friend. Staying active and busy is absolutely my best dieting trick.

Slow down. Let time be your biggest asset. By eating at a leisurely pace, you give your body the twenty minutes it needs to recognize that it has been fed. Enjoy each bite. Put your fork down frequently and talk. Sit and sip your coffee or tea slowly. In the long run, you'll eat less.

Stay satisfied. Follow your food plan and be sated with each day's food. And be thankful for it. In our country, the motto is more, more, more! Your body only needs so much food each day. Anything over that is surplus. (Think of it like your bank account. There's only so much money in there.

If you write more checks than money, it's against the law!)
Recruit the Holy Spirit to help you "just say no."

It's so hard, isn't it? Watch TV for five minutes and you'll
see three fast-food commercials. You didn't even have to
leave your sofa to be tempted by visuals of mouth-watering
hamburgers dripping all over the place, good-and-greasy
fries, pulse-quickening pizzas, sugary fruit-flavored cereals that even come with a prize, addictive sodas, soothing
chocolate candy bars, and cheesy nachos sizzling with spice.
Makes you want to take a run to the border, doesn't it? Like
Pavlov's dog, we're conditioned to salivate at the next commercial. Oh, the ways of the world . . . so many temptations.
The Bible contains wisdom for our food intake: Enjoy what
God has given us within the boundaries he has set. Use
moderation. Stay self-controlled. Stay Spirit-controlled,
not network-controlled.

Stick by your standard. Another way I (Cynthia) control
my weight is to hold to a standard. I have a maximum weight
that I allow myself to climb to, but I won't go over that. I
tell my husband, "I'm right at the line again. If I go over, I
start to look fat." He always reassures me, "You don't look fat
. . ." That gives me at least another week of overeating before
I'm forced to face reality. I like this little game. But when I
hit the max, I cut back on calories. I watch my food intake
throughout the week. If we splurge on the weekends, then
I reduce my meals on Monday, Tuesday, and Wednesday
(or whatever it takes). If I eat breakfast out and overdo,
then I don't eat the rest of the day and have soup for supper.
We all know it's easier to lose three pounds than thirty. I
call this "the three-pound solution." Maintenance is easier
than overhaul!

A Whole New World

You are learning a whole new way of eating for a whole new you. As you establish a better pattern of diet and exercise, your life will improve. Slothful living doesn't satisfy. Energetic activity, accomplishments, and relationships do. Junk diets don't satisfy either. In a study at the University of Alabama, subjects were allowed as much as they desired from a whole foods diet like the *Healthy Balance* diet. They were also offered as much as it took for gratification on refined, processed foods. With whole foods, it took 1500 calories to be satisfied, but it took over 3000 calories before the subjects stopped eating the junk. Dr. Howard Shapiro demonstrates this visually on pages 4–5 of his beautiful book *Picture Perfect Weight Loss*. The first page shows a breakfast muffin worth 720 calories. Now that's one monster muffin! But look what you can get for the same amount of calories . . .

The next page illustrates the amount of whole foods you can get for 720 calories: 2 small whole-wheat rolls, 2 pears, some green grapes, ½ papaya, ½ kiwi, ½ cantaloupe, and 1 whole pineapple! And look at all the colors you're consuming! The *Healthy Balance* program is such a satisfying way to eat.

The world offers us junk food spiritually too. Trashy, silly TV programs, shallow literature, sensual music, senseless chatter, time wasters—these will never satisfy. We were made for the deep mysteries of life. Only Jesus Christ will meet the profound needs of the human heart.

The article "Soul Food," excerpted from Dr. Charles Stanley's monthly magazine *In Touch,* confirms the satisfaction of knowing the Savior.

As a Christian, you must exercise great care in regard to your appetites. Although the world offers many tantalizing choices, these things bring only temporary pleasure, leaving behind a feeling of emptiness. For example, the desire to marry or enjoy a successful career is not sinful in itself, but you should be careful not to allow any person or thing to take the place of Christ in your life. In other words, you must guard your God-given appetites so they will not be twisted or perverted by the Enemy.

In order to combat worldly "hungers," you must receive the proper spiritual nourishment. Walking with the Lord will satisfy your appetite with His Word, and quench your soul's thirst with His living water. Your needs will only be satisfied by the Creator.[5]

Healthy Balance secret #2: Practice moderation in all things.

God has an answer for our souls' deepest cravings: daily intake of his Word and satisfying times in communication with him. He also has an answer for weight control: high-quality, satisfying, naturally low-fat foods and biblical self-control.

5

Recipes
for a Healthy Balance

We haven't found any other eating plan as satisfying as the *Healthy Balance* way. The variety, the fresh whole foods, the simplicity . . . God had a great plan in mind at Creation. Nutritious eating has become second nature to us. And it will be the same for you when you add some of these cooking tips and recipes to your repertoire. Your kitchen is stocked with delicious, wholesome foods. Fresh fruit is on your table. Seeds and nuts are on hand for snacking, and grains and legumes are in the pantry. The produce is washed and stored in the frig. The butter is softened and the beans are soaking. Let's get cooking!

Healthy Balance Cookery

Steaming. Cooking the *Healthy Balance* way is so simple because your meals are simple. Steaming is one of the most nutritious cooking methods that we've found. It's an easy way to make your *Healthy Balance* meal. Toss the food portions into a steamer basket, your protein, whole grains and legumes first (all previously cooked), then your variety of vegetables. Don't forget the garlic and onion for seasoning!

Suspend the steamer basket above a covered pot of boiling water until the vegetables are lightly steamed. If you are cooking for a family, increase the portions. Vegetables vary in steaming time from five to twenty-five minutes, so check their texture frequently. Remove and season to taste. Kelp powder, sea salt, nutritional yeast, plain pepper, cayenne pepper, ginger, curry, and other spices add flavor. Vinegar, lemon juice, mustard, sodium-free soy sauce, or Bragg's Amino Acids are good too. Olive oil and Balanced Butter can be used in moderation (if you are weight reducing, be sure to count them as your daily fat, however).

Sauteing. You can also cook your meat or poultry separately, dry sauteing it (or using a fat-free spray) in a nonstick skillet. Then steam your vegetables of choice.

Stir-frying. It's nearly as quick and just as nutrient-dense as steaming. First, prepare your sauce:

Stir-Fry Sauce

In a bowl combine:

¼ cup fat-free chicken broth, ½ cup orange juice, 2 Tbs soy sauce, 1 Tbs grated fresh ginger, 1 tsp sesame oil, 1 Tbs cornstarch (optional: 1 Tbs sugar or honey)

Set aside to use in stir-fry.

Then dice your protein (1 pound of beef, poultry, pork, or seafood, or ⅔ pound meat, ⅓ pound tofu) into ½-inch cubes. Chop a colorful array of vegetables: onions or scallions, carrots, celery, cauliflower, broccoli, your favorites. Shred some cabbage and mince a head of garlic. Pour 2 Tbs of olive oil into your nonstick skillet and first saute your protein portions for five minutes or so until done. Add the chopped veggies and saute two minutes. Next add the cabbage, garlic, and prepared sauce. Stir as you fry, around three minutes. If sauce thickens too much, thin with water. Place a lid over the pan, turn off the burner, and allow the food to steam while dishing up plates with precooked brown rice. This stir-fry is good over the top of any whole grain.

Grilling. In the summer, cook your complete meal outdoors. Throw some shrimp on the barbie. But also marinate some vegetables like red and green bell peppers, corn on the cob, potatoes, tomatoes, zucchini, or even hot peppers. Lay them on the grill during the last few minutes of cook time. Serve with a refreshing salad and some iced green tea.

Baking. Winter baking and roasting is another healthy alternative. Brown your meat or chicken, both sides, in some fat-free spray. Lay in the bottom of a Pyrex dish. Layer potatoes, carrots, onions, minced garlic, turnips, celery on top. Any of your favorite vegetables will do, but root vegetables roast especially well. Salt and pepper and cover with foil. Bake at 350 degrees for one hour. The juices and flavors of the meat and vegetables blend, creating a delicious but easy dish.

In the summer, don't heat up the house. You can also arrange the same ingredients (except for the potatoes) in a crockpot before leaving for work. The food must cook at least five hours on high or eight hours on low. Often we'll omit the meat or poultry and just bake or roast a whole pan of vegetables drizzled with olive oil and sprinkled with minced garlic and sea salt. The above vegetables work well for this idea, as do winter squash. Bake some prescrubbed yams and sweet potatoes ahead in your oven or crockpot and keep them bagged in the frig. You can microwave them for a quick meal or a snack. Nothing tastes better than a roasted yam or sweet potato sprinkled with sea salt and moistened with Balanced Butter. Yum! It's the perfect dessert on a cold winter evening.

Juicing. Freshly made juice is a fantastic way to get your fruits and veggies for the day. You can drink the juice as it comes from the plant within the first ten minutes before the enzymes begin to oxidize. Or you can pour the fruit juice into a blender, add soy powder or yogurt, maybe a frozen banana or a cup of berries, five cubes of ice, and you have a smoothie. We use a juicer for fruit and vegetable juices, but we also both own Vita-Mix machines. These machines are among our most valuable kitchen equipment—they do everything in a matter of minutes. Chop, dice, shred, puree, blend. Make soup, bread, even nutritious "ice cream" out of fruits. The health advantage of the Vita-Mix is that the cell walls of the fresh, whole foods are ruptured, making their phytonutrients more available to the body. Also, the fiber is retained in the soup or drink. The Vita-Mix is easy to use and just as easy to clean. The machine makes whole meals as simple as a flip of a switch. In your kitchen, you need a few appliances to assist you in making healthy meals. For more information about Vita-Mix machines, you can check our web site, www.lifebalanceladies.com.

> The discovery of a new dish is more beneficial to humanity than the discovery of a new star.
>
> Anthelme Brillat-Savarin
> (1755–1826)

Juices and smoothies are quick ways to get your nutrition when you're in a morning rush. Breakfast can also be any of the meals above (leftovers heat up quickly) or an omelette packed with veggies and chased down with some fresh vitamin-rich juice. Oatmeal with nonfat milk and some fruit is great in the morning, or toast with no-sugar fruit preserves or nut butter (count the fat) and coffee. Or try a nutritious packaged breakfast shake. Eating a good breakfast will boost your metabolism for the day. You've been fasting all night, and your body needs food for energy.

Healthy Balance Cooking

A Salad a Day . . .

A *Healthy Balance* salad is a cool, delicious way to enjoy your fresh veggies. Plus the enzymes in the raw foods aid digestion. Have a fresh, raw salad every day to ensure your body gets the enzymes it needs for absorption of nutrients. Using the suggested vegetables in the color categories, chop each category into bite-sized pieces, tear the greens, and toss with lemon or vinegar and olive oil. Another favorite dressing is Marie's Blue Cheese or Creamy Italian (made with whole ingredients, but minus the sugar that other dressings have). Several of Paul Newman's dressings are also sugar-free. Check the labels. You can include your protein in your salad: hard-boiled egg, pieces of fish or tuna, meat or poultry, legumes (see recipes that follow). Serve your grain as some delicious fresh bread on the side.

The Healthy Balance Salad

Toss together in large salad bowl:

2 cups of romaine and other leafy lettuces, washed, dried, and torn into pieces

2 cups spinach, collard greens, or kale, washed, dried, and torn into small pieces

½ cup chopped yellow squash or pepper, ½ cup grated sweet potato or carrot

½ cup chopped red onion, 1 cup chopped broccoli, 1 cup shredded red cabbage

½ cup chopped mushrooms, celery, or cauliflower

½ cup brown rice or other grain cooked with almonds

1 cup cooked legumes

Store in refrigerator.

Serve with balsamic vinegar and extra-virgin olive oil. (Or try one of our dressing recipes below.)

The Ever-Ready Healthy Balance *Salad Bar*

It helps me (Charity) to always keep a "salad bar" ready in my refrigerator. When I come home from a modeling shoot or audition, I'm usually starving. I'll grab a bowl and fill it with salad goodies that I've prepared in advance. Here's my secret to successful and healthy weight maintenance:

Bring your fresh produce home from the market and immediately wash and dry it. Soak the leafy greens in a vegetable wash, scrub the carrots and turnips, wash the green vegetables. Rinse and dry. I throw the leafy greens like lettuce, kale, and chard into a salad spinner. This removes excess water and keeps greens fresh longer. Tear the lettuce and greens into bite-sized pieces and store in baggies in the frig.

Now you're ready to chop, slice, and dice your other veggies into a colorful rainbow of salad-ready toppings. Carrots, celery, cucumbers, radishes, jicama, bell pepper (red and green), broccoli, and cauliflower are some of my favorites.

Shred some low-fat cheese like mozzarella or feta. Chop some nuts, almonds, or pecans. If you like a little sweetness in your salad, you can also include raisins, cranberries, or other dried fruits. Sectioned citrus like oranges and grapefruit mix well with green salads. And of course avocados, but don't eat too many of them while on a weight loss plan. Although their oils are good for us, the fat still has too many calories for losing weight. Canned beans can be drained and added to your salads for fat-free protein and flavor.

After the chopping is finished, you can put each category of food in its own small plasticware container or baggie in the frig. It helps to keep these containers on a tray on the refrigerator shelf to pull out at a moment's notice. Just as easily, you can put them back to store for the next meal. Now you have your own salad bar ready when you are!

Somewhere over the Rainbow

In the winter, most of us crave something warm. I (Cynthia) like warm foods any time of year! Charity's salad idea has helped me stay on the *Healthy Balance* nutrition plan, but it also helps to keep some healthy soups ready to heat up. Here's a simple recipe:

The *Healthy Balance* Simply Super Soup

Dice and slice your favorite vegetables and add a cooked protein (don't forget legumes are a protein!).

Toss them all into a pot of vegetable broth.

Simmer mixture for fifteen minutes, and enjoy!

You can add your grain to the soup when you season, or serve it as a bread accompaniment.

As kids we were told, "Follow the rainbow and you'll find your pot of gold." Today's "pot of gold" may well be a soup pot. As we've discussed, scientists are now discovering what God told us way back in the beginning: *Vegetables are the key to good health.* Fresh, low-fat plant foods are unequaled in preventing disease and obesity. And for most of us, nothing is heartier than a big bowl of steaming vegetable soup.

Studies indicate that people who enjoy soup before meals eat less and lose more weight. Author Barbara Rolls, Ph.D., a professor at Pennsylvania State University, tested twenty-four college students. On three separate days, the women were instructed to choose between a small portion of chicken rice casserole, an equal portion of casserole plus a large glass of water, or a big bowl of chicken rice soup (which had the same ingredients as the casserole plus the same amount of water, 10 oz, as the glass). Seventeen minutes later, lunch was served, a full buffet featuring ham and cheese, kaiser rolls, lettuces, tomato and cucumber slices, chips, pretzels, fruit-flavored yogurt, cookies, and chocolate candy bars. They were ordered to eat as much as they wanted. (Any volunteers for that study?) The casserole eaters, with or without the water accompaniment, chose lunches equaling 400 calories. Amazingly, the soup eaters ate only 300 calories. At dinner, the consumption for the soup eaters didn't increase. Again, the calorie count rose to only 300.[1] Make your soup a hearty vegetable and you'll not only decrease calories, you'll increase your colors!

My secret for staying on the *Healthy Balance* eating plan is to make a big pot of vegetable soup once or twice a week and eat that before (or in place of) meals. I usually make a crockpot of beans too. That way, I ingest the different categories of vegetables quickly and easily because they are prepared ahead. In addition, soup is easier for a sick person to digest, and I was trying to get well when I began this program.

Usually lunch consists of a bowl of soup and Charity's big tossed salad recipe of torn leafy greens loaded with crunchy, diced vegetables. I might put my protein into the salad or serve it on the side. One other suggestion: Don't mix tomatoes into your salad until ready to serve. And don't store other foods with tomatoes—they make everything soggy! Put them in their own container.

I'll usually have a bowl of soup before dinner and sometimes even before breakfast. Once or twice a week, I'll eat beans for breakfast. I'm craving something warm and filling, but I'm also usually in a rush. Prepared foods are quick to heat up!

Here are my personal recipes for soup stocks and several soup variations:

Beef Stock

Brown 2-pound roast (or bones with meat on them) in oven at 450 degrees for 45 minutes.

Add 4 quartered onions with skin on, a garlic bulb cut in half, 2 chopped carrots, 3 stalks celery including tops, and 1 quartered turnip.

Roast at 450 degrees for 1 additional hour.

Place all in stockpot after pouring off fat. Cover with pure water. Toss in 2 bay leaves, salt (2 tsp) and pepper (1 tsp), and favorite herbs like rosemary or thyme.

Bring to a boil, then simmer for half a day. (Can also be made in crockpot on high.)

Remove meat after 1 hour. (You can cool this meat, shred, and freeze for tacos or casseroles later.)

Toss bones back into pot. Cook quickly.

Strain vegetables and remove fat (with fat separator, frozen cheesecloth, or by cooling broth to let fat rise to the top to be skimmed off).

Chicken Stock

Roast a whole, cleaned chicken in your crockpot or oven. Salt and pepper the inside of the chicken before roasting and stuff chopped onion and garlic inside.

Add root vegetables as in beef stock (but no rosemary or thyme).

When chicken is roasted and browned (about 1 hour in oven, 350 degrees, or in crockpot on high for 5 hours), cool. Pull meat off and save (can be frozen for later, used in your salad that day or the next, or plan tacos that night!).

Set aside meat juices. Put bones in pot and cover with water.

Bring to a boil, then turn down heat, add juices from crockpot, and simmer for 2 more hours.

Strain, discard vegetables, and run broth through a fat separator. Or chill in frig and skim off fat. Cool. (Broth can be frozen now for future use or set aside for soup.)

You can also stew a chicken on the stovetop for broth:

Stovetop Chicken Stock

Wash a chicken well. Place breast side up in large pot.

Cover chicken with pure water.

Toss in some vegetables and seasoning. (I usually add a carrot or two, some celery stalks and leaves, chopped onion, minced garlic, maybe a turnip, some stems left-over from greens. I save everything for these healthy broths!) Most vegetables work well except broccoli and bell pepper. (These vegetables give it a distinctive and not always pleasant taste.)

Salt and pepper. Bring to a boil, then simmer for 1 hour.

Remove chicken. Cool and take meat from bone.

Throw bones back into stockpot and simmer another 2 hours.

Pour everything through a colander into another pot. Discard the bones and veggies.

The broth in the pot can be poured through a fat separator or cooled in the frig until the fat rises to the top and can be skimmed off.

You can also make a vegetarian broth by eliminating the chicken:

Vegan Broth

Toss the vegetables listed above into a pot filled with pure water.

Simmer for 1 hour.

Strain. Season to taste.

Now that you have your broth on hand, you're ready to make your hearty soup:

Cynthia's *Healthy Balance* Chicken Soup

In a pot on the stove, sauté:

1 chopped onion and 2–3 large minced garlic cloves in 1 Tbs of olive oil

Add defatted broth.

Chop 2–3 carrots, 2 small turnips, 2–3 stalks celery, 1 peeled tomato, 1 cup of cauliflower, 1 zucchini, and other produce that appeals to you. (I only use broccoli stalks as the florets give the soup a sharp taste. No bell pepper either.)

Add to broth and simmer 30 minutes.

The last 10 minutes of cooking time, add ½ small head of cabbage, shredded, or 1 cup of shredded kale or collard greens. Simmer. (Remember, gauge the amount of vegetables carefully—you do want broth in your soup. If there isn't enough liquid, add water and a couple of chicken bouillon cubes or a large can of fat-free chicken broth.)

Season to taste.

Makes a large pot. Can feed a family of five two nights or one hungry woman several days!

Serve with some whole-grain bread or rolls spread with the healthiest "butter" you've ever tasted!

Soup Variations:

1. Dice cooked chicken and add to soup just before serving. Or noodles can be added the last 10 minutes when you add the greens.

2. During last 10 minutes of cooking, spoon in a small can of bean with bacon soup. Also, add 1 can of water. Simmer until greens are cooked and serve.

3. When soup is finished (vegetable soup only), puree the whole pot in a blender. Makes a creamy, green soup. Season to taste and serve.

Balanced Butter

Place in a Vita-Mix, blender, or bowl:

1 cup softened butter, 1 cup extra-virgin olive oil or flax-seed oil (which has a slightly different taste; found in health stores). Or you can use ½ cup olive oil and ½ cup flaxseed oil.

Blend (or mix with mixer) thoroughly. Will be slightly runny.

Spoon into storage container and refrigerate.

Balanced Butter solidifies when cooled but remains spreadable.

Balanced Butter Variations:

1. Garlic Butter: If you like garlic butter for your whole-grain French bread, place some of the butter mixture in a small sealable container. Mix in garlic salt or garlic powder. You can also use roasted garlic or even raw minced garlic.

2. Honey or Fruit Butter: Reduce olive oil to ½ cup. Add ½ cup of warmed honey or sugar-free fruit preserves. Mix together with 1 cup of softened butter. Refrigerate. Spread it on whole-grain toast, rolls, or biscuits when you want a tasty, wholesome treat for your family.

Balanced Butter provides the benefits of the Omega-3 fatty acids found in good oils. My kids love it as much as I (Cynthia) do. Plus my dinner guests praise me as if I'm Martha Stewart. When my kids tell their friends Mom made it, visitors exclaim, "What? You even make your own butter!" Smug smile from the chef's corner . . .

Beans, Beans, the Musical Fruit

I (Cynthia) always thought this childhood poem was so creative—it had such a great rhyming rhythm to it! But there is also a lot of truth to the ditty. If beans aren't prepared correctly, they can bloat you up like the Goodyear Blimp. That's why many people stay away from them. But the other truth is that they are really nutritious. The more you eat, the better you will feel. I don't recommend them for every meal, as the poem suggests, but I aim for some legumes, cooked right, every day. Here is my favorite recipe:

Cynthia's *Balance* Beans

Wash and drain 2 cups of small white beans. Great Northerns are terrific, as are Cannellinis. Discard any rocks, blackened beans, and the like.

Place beans in a large pot and cover with water. Soak all night. Drain. Or if making the same day, cover with water and bring to a boil. Turn off heat and let sit for 2 hours. Drain.

In large pot, saute for 2 minutes in 1–2 Tbs olive oil with a chopped onion, several cloves of minced garlic, 2–3 diced carrots, 2–3 stalks diced celery and some leaves. Optional: Add 1 peeled, diced turnip at this point. Remember, any vegetables you add to recipes will benefit your health. Avoid strong-flavored veggies here, though.

Add the drained beans. Cover all with pure water or your chicken or vegetable broth. I usually use the chicken broth for extra flavor, either my own or fat-free canned if I'm in a hurry.

Bring to a boil for 2 minutes. Then simmer for 2 hours (do not boil, because beans will burst) until beans are the consistency that you prefer. I personally favor soft beans. A half hour before serving, season with salt and pepper to taste. Optional seasonings are a small pinch of curry, cumin, or celery seed, only one though. The simpler the taste, the better! You don't want to add the salt until the last half hour of cooking. Salt will toughen the beans if added before this point. (I often use a crockpot for beans.)

2 cups of dried beans makes 4 to 6 cups cooked.

Bean Variations:

1. For ham-flavored beans, add a ham bone and 1 tsp of smoke flavoring to the recipe above.

2. In the last 5 minutes of cooking, add ½ head of green cabbage, shredded.

Charity Chats

Mom uses soup before many of her meals to curb her appetite. I'm often in a hurry with no time to make soup (although canned low-fat works just as well!). But, I have my own secret weapon: Eat an apple about twenty minutes before your meal. The fiber fills you up and the pectin in the fruit controls your appetite. Yet an apple is fat-free with only about 85 calories for a medium-sized fruit.

You know how legend has it that an apple tempted Adam and Eve . . . well, an apple can keep you from temptation when it comes to the buffet table! The really cool thing is there are over 2400 varieties of apples, so you'll never be bored. Try a different one before each meal. An apple a day keeps the pounds away!

Balance Beans with Chili

For spicy beans, south-of-the-border: Use pintos, navies, or cranberry beans. Prepare as above plus throw in 1 diced bell pepper and 2 peeled tomatoes.

Add 1 can tomato sauce, 1 tsp oregano, ½ tsp ground cumin, 1 tsp or more powdered chili (depending on your taste).

Simmer and serve with heated tortillas.

The *Healthy Balance* salad, soup, and beans are the standbys that keep us on our nutritious eating plan in these hectic, busy days. Keep them in your refrigerator and see if that helps you stay balanced too!

Additional Recipes

Pam Wolfenbarger, Cynthia's sister, is a great cook. We've borrowed two of our favorite recipes from her. Here is a quick, complete meal with an Oriental flavor for the whole family to enjoy. Eri, our exchange student from Japan, loved to eat it with chopsticks when she stayed with the Allens. (Watch for our upcoming LifeBalance series book *The Healthy Balance Cookbook*. We'll have more easy, tasty treats like the ones that follow for you and your family!)

Pam's Yaki Soba

Brown 1 pound of lean ground beef (or saute skinless cubed chicken in 1 Tbs olive oil) and drain.

While stirring, add 2–3 cloves minced garlic, 1 Tbs ginger, ¼ cup chopped green onions, 2–3 shredded carrots, and ½ of a green cabbage, shredded. (Or you can buy the packaged, preshredded coleslaw mix.)

Mix ¼ cup soy sauce with ¼ cup water and pour over meat/vegetable mixture.

While vegetables are cooking, prepare 3 packages of ramen noodles according to directions, but don't add the flavor packets. Drain the noodles and add to the meat mixture.

Add more soy sauce if needed, and any other favorite seasonings.

Pam's Authentic Salsa

In Vita-Mix or blender combine:

2 large cans peeled tomatoes, 1 onion, 1 bell pepper, 1–6 large cloves of garlic, 1 bunch of cilantro, 8–10 serrano or jalapeno chilies, 1 or 1½ tsp salt (or salt to taste)

Whirl briefly until vegetables are blended, but don't reduce to a liquid.

Fantastic to serve with tortilla chips, of course. But for the dieter, use with celery, bell pepper, and jicama slices. Or pour over scrambled eggs or a baked potato. Also use as fat-free dressing for tostadas and salads.

Tricolor Omelette

Spray small nonstick skillet with fat-free spray.

Saute ⅛ cup chopped onions, ⅛ cup chopped bell pepper, ⅛ cup chopped tomato or mushrooms.

While veggies are cooking, mix 1 egg and 2 whites.

Remove cooked vegetables onto plate. Pour egg mixture into pan.

Tilt skillet to cover bottom with mixture. Lift omelette occasionally to allow mixture to set. Salt and pepper to taste.

Slide omelette onto plate, fill with vegetables, and fold.

Makes 1 serving.

Traditional Oatmeal

In saucepan, bring 1½ cups water to a boil.

Add ½ tsp salt and 1 tsp cinnamon.

Stir in ¾ cup old-fashioned oatmeal and allow to simmer 5 minutes, until thickened.

Serve with sweetener or brown sugar, 1 percent milk or almond milk, and condiments like raisins, chopped nuts, or diced apple.

Fruit Smoothies

In Vita-Mix or blender place:

1 cup nonfat milk (soy, almond, or dairy), 1½ cups frozen berries, sugar-free (strawberries, raspberries, or blueberries), ½ frozen banana, ¼ cup light tofu, 1 tsp sweetener, sugar, or honey

Run on high for 30 seconds, then add:

2 cups frozen strawberries, 6 oz unsweetened pineapple juice,
1 tsp vanilla extract, 5 oz tofu, firm or extra firm, 3 Tbs honey (optional), 1 Tbs coconut juice or flavoring (optional)

Run on high for 30 seconds.

Makes 2 servings. Enjoy!

Vegetable Juice

With juicer or Vita-Mix, juice:

3 carrots, 2 stalks of celery, ½ beet, 1 cucumber, handful of greens (kale, collards, cabbage)

Makes one tall glass of fresh juice containing 9 servings of vegetables. (The Vita-Mix juice is thicker with more pulp and more fiber.)

Crunchy Coleslaw

In Vita-Mix container place:

1 small cabbage cut in wedges (about 4 cups), 1 cup carrots, ½ red onion, 2 celery stalks.

Fill the container with water and secure lid. Set on high speed and quickly turn machine off and on 3–4 times until vegetables are chopped.

Don't overprocess. Drain well, pressing out liquid.

Hand method: Shred with a knife or grate cabbage, carrots, red onion, and celery.

Place shredded veggies in bowl and mix with following dressing.

Coleslaw Dressing

In Vita-Mix or blender, mix:

½ cup nonfat mayonnaise, ½ cup fat-free sour cream, ½ tsp salt,½ tsp apple cider vinegar, pepper, and sweetener (optional) to taste.

Makes 9 almost fat-free ½ cup servings.

Low-fat Italian Dressing

Mix in Vita-Mix or shake in covered container:

½ cup olive oil, ½ cup apple juice, ¼ cup white wine vinegar, 2 Tbs finely chopped onion, 1 tsp dried basil, ½ tsp dried oregano, ½ tsp salt, ¼ tsp pepper, 2–3 cloves minced garlic (your preference)

Store in frig and shake before serving.

Dressing Variations:

1. Creamy Italian: Blend until smooth ½ cup Italian dressing with ½ cup low-fat mayonnaise. Store in refrigerator.

2. Parmesan Garlic: To Italian dressing recipe, add ¼ cup finely grated low-fat Parmesan cheese. Shake well before serving.

Corn Bread

In Vita-Mix or blender:

Blend ¾ cup water, 1 egg or 2 egg whites, ¼ cup canola oil, ¾ cup plain fat-free yogurt, 2 Tbs sugar-free peach or apricot jam.

Fold in gently to moisten: 1 cup unbleached flour, 2 Tbs toasted wheat germ, 1½ cups cornmeal, 4 tsp baking powder, ½ tsp salt.

Pour into square pan coated with nonstick cooking spray.

Bake at 400 degrees for 15–20 minutes until browned.

Serve with Balanced Butter.

Baked Vegetables

Spray 9 x 11 Pyrex dish with nonstick spray.

Lay washed vegetables in sections of pan: red potatoes, carrots, turnips, mushrooms (another time try winter squash, sweet potatoes, or yams).

Sprinkle with salt and pepper.

Layer quartered onions and minced garlic over the top of the vegetables and drizzle with olive oil.

Cover with foil. Bake at 350 degrees for 1 hour.

Variation: Make a one-dish meal. Bottom layer browned, seasoned chicken breasts; middle layer red potatoes, carrots, turnips, mushrooms, salt and pepper; top layer quartered onions, minced garlic, olive oil. Cover with foil. Bake at 350 degrees for 1 hour.

Skinny Mashed Potatoes

Peel 6 medium potatoes and place in pot. Cover with salted water.

Toss in some chopped garlic for flavor.

Boil for 30–35 minutes until soft, then drain.

In bowl mash until no lumps remain, mixing in heated fat-free chicken broth until mashed potatoes are preferred consistency.

Salt and pepper to taste. Place dollop of Balanced Butter in the center.

Makes 4 servings.

Italian Chicken and Cheese Calzones

Preheat oven to 375 degrees. Spray a baking sheet with nonstick cooking spray and dust with cornmeal.

Coat a nonstick skillet with cooking spray and saute 1 thinly sliced onion over medium heat.

After 5–7 minutes, stir in ¾ pound cooked, shredded chicken (can use the chicken left over from making soup stock).

Add 1 cup canned spaghetti sauce.

Mix in ¼ cup vegetables (grated zucchini or bell pepper) and 2 Tbs chopped olives. Heat through.

Open 2 tubes of refrigerated pizza dough (10 oz each). On lightly floured breadboard, divide into 4 equal pieces. Roll 1 piece of dough into a 7-inch circle.

Place ½ cup of chicken mixture on top of circle; spread to 1 inch of edge. Sprinkle with ¼ cup of grated low-fat mozzarella cheese.

Brush the edges of the crust with an egg-white mixture (1 egg white, lightly beaten with 1 tsp water). Fold the circle in half and pinch edges to seal.

Repeat with dough and filling to make 4 calzones total.

Place on prepared baking sheet. Brush calzones with egg-white mixture. With sharp knife, make 3 tiny slashes on top of each calzone.

Bake for 20–25 minutes until crusts are golden brown. Cut each calzone in half and serve.

Roasted Garlic Chicken with Vegetables

Wash and dry 2-pound or 3-pound chicken. Place in 9 x 11 Pyrex dish sprayed with nonstick spray.

Rub salt, pepper, garlic powder, and favorite seasonings inside cavity of chicken.

Lay peeled carrots, onions, and potatoes (enough for your family), all quartered, alongside the chicken.

Salt, pepper, and season. Sprinkle top of all with 2–3 cloves of minced garlic.

Cover with foil. Bake for 1 hour at 350 degrees.

Remove vegetables to serving platter.

Bake chicken without foil for 10 more minutes to brown top. Transfer to serving platter.

Colorful Crustless Quiche

Preheat oven to 400 degrees. Spray 10-inch pie dish with cooking spray.

Mix in large bowl: 2 cups egg substitute or egg mixture (1 cup whole eggs, about 5, and 1 cup egg whites, about 10—save the yolks for the kids' French toast the next morning), ⅓ cup flour, 1 tsp baking powder, 6 oz nonfat cottage cheese, ½ package (10 oz) frozen chopped spinach (thawed and liquid squeezed out), ½ cup filled with thinly sliced green onions and mushrooms, grated carrots, red bell pepper (or colorful veggies of choice). Stir in ¼ tsp cayenne pepper, ¼ tsp salt, ⅛ tsp pepper.

Pour into pie dish and bake 15 minutes.

Lower heat to 350 degrees and bake 35–40 minutes longer until filling is set. Insert toothpick to check doneness. When toothpick comes out clean, quiche is done.

Cool on a rack 10 minutes before serving.

Serves 6–8.

Marinated Steak

Combine in 9 x 11 Pyrex dish:

2 cups soy sauce, 2 Tbs brown sugar, 3 minced cloves garlic, 1 tsp coarse black pepper

Lay 4 steaks in marinade, then turn over. Cover with plastic wrap and refrigerate.

Marinate 4 hours or more, turning occasionally.

Remove steaks from marinade, scraping off garlic bits and pepper.

Grill, broil, or panfry to desired doneness.

Vegi-Grain Saute

Melt 2 tsp Balanced Butter in skillet over medium-high heat.

Cook 1 chopped large onion (1 cup), 1 medium chopped yellow or red bell pepper (1 cup), and 1 crushed garlic clove in butter until done (about 2 minutes; bell pepper should still be slightly crisp).

Stir in 4 cups cooked brown rice or barley, 2 tsp dried thyme leaves, ½ tsp salt, 1 package frozen corn, thawed, 1 package frozen lima beans, thawed.

Cook until heated through.

Makes 4 servings of 2 cups, each with 360 calories and 3 grams fat.

The *Healthy Balance* Italian Style

I (Charity) love Italian food! Here are several recipes I've created that quench my cravings but don't pile on the pounds.

Charity's Italian Vegi-Bake

Preheat oven to 350 degrees. Spray 9 x 12 x 2 baking pan with nonstick spray.

Cut in round slices 1 eggplant, 2 green peppers, 1 onion, 4 tomatoes, mushrooms, broccoli, and carrots.

Layer some of vegetables to cover bottom of pan.

Sprinkle grated low-fat mozzarella over first layer (about ⅔ cup per layer).

Continue to layer veggies and cheese. Sprinkle top layer of veggies with cheese.

Pour 1 can spaghetti sauce (16 oz) over entire casserole.

Cover with foil and bake for 1 hour.

Serves 4 as a side dish. For a complete meal, add diced cooked chicken or cooked lean ground beef to layers and bake as directed.

Guilt-free Pasta with Vegetable Cream Sauce

In saucepan, mix 1 tsp cornstarch and 1 tsp nonfat milk.

Add 1 can evaporated skim milk and 1–2 cloves of minced garlic.

Stir as mixture comes to a boil.

Lower heat and stir while adding 8 oz fat-free cream cheese.

(Can also add thawed bagged peas/carrots combo for more color.)

Simmer mixture until thick. Salt and pepper to taste.

Saute ⅓ pound sliced mushrooms and 4 chopped green onions in skillet coated with nonstick spray. Add to cream sauce.

Cook pasta (fettucini or angel hair are nice) per package directions. Drain pasta and top with sauce. (Sauce can also be served over brown rice, baked potatoes, cooked vegetables, or meat dishes.) Yum!

Meatless Italian Sauce

Heat 2 Tbs olive oil in 3-quart saucepan over medium heat.

Saute in oil 1 large chopped onion, 1 medium chopped green bell pepper, and 3 minced cloves of garlic.

Stir in 2 cans whole tomatoes (16 oz), 2 cans tomato sauce (8 oz), 2 tsp dried basil, 1 tsp dried oregano, ¾ tsp salt, ¼ tsp pepper.

Bring to boil, breaking up tomatoes while stirring. Reduce to low and simmer for 45 minutes or until desired consistency.

Serve over pasta, brown rice, baked potatoes, or meat dishes.

Charity's Raspberry Refresher

Bring 5 cups water to a boil.

Place 3 fruit-flavored herbal tea bags in a heat-proof pitcher.

Pour hot water over tea bags, allowing to steep for 4–5 minutes.

Remove tea bags, cover and refrigerate until cool (20–30 minutes).

In Vita-Mix, blend thawed, unsweetened frozen raspberries (or other berries) until smooth.

Strain puree and add to pitcher of tea. Stir in sugar substitute equivalent (to ⅓ cup sugar), 1 tsp lemon juice, and ice cubes to chill. Stir, pour into tall glasses, and enjoy!

Fat-free Heavenly Dessert

Tear 1 angel food cake (preferably day-old) into pieces and arrange in dessert bowl.

Prepare 2 small boxes sugar-free Jell-O (favorite flavor. Charity's is strawberry-banana) according to directions. Keep the Jell-O liquid, however. Don't gel in frig.

Pour the liquid Jell-O mixture over the cake pieces in bowl. With large spoon, gently toss cake around in Jell-O mixture until the liquid is absorbed into the cake. Cover and place bowl in refrigerator until Jell-O sets well. Top dessert with lite whipped topping before serving.

159 calories per serving. A fat-free treat for 8 guests.

Pudding Parfaits Pronto

Combine in small bowl: 1 cup skim milk, or nonfat half and half, 8 oz nonfat yogurt (a fruit flavor), 1 small package instant, fat-free, sugar-free vanilla pudding.

Beat until thickened, 2 minutes on low speed.

Prepare 2–3 cups fresh fruit (strawberries and bananas, or pineapple and bananas)

In six parfait glasses, arrange alternating layers of fruit and pudding mixtures, beginning with fruit at bottom.

Chill. Garnish with fruit slices before serving.

Out to Lunch

America eats out almost as much as at home. Research shows that women who eat out often, around six times a week, consume 288 more calories and 19 more grams of fat per day than those who eat out five times a week or less.[2] That can add up to a whopping 25 pounds gained per year! Restaurant meals make it hard to stay balanced on a healthy eating plan. The restaurant dishes are laden with hidden fats and sugars. The plates are large enough to hold a Thanksgiving turkey. And most importantly, there's a tendency to try to eat as much as possible because "I paid for it." Besides, the food is usually really, really good! (They aim for that—it keeps customers rolling in. After all, who keeps visiting a restaurant that serves nasty food!)

> The destiny of nations depends on the manner wherein they take their food.
>
> Anthelme Brillat-Savarin (1755–1826)

You can have your restaurant food and eat it too, however. Adhere to a few rules when you go out and you won't destroy any progress you've made in your weight loss program.

Stick to low-fat meals.

Request that food be prepared these ways: roasted, poached, steamed, grilled, broiled, and stir-fried. Ask the waiter to leave off gravies, sauces, and butters. (Carry along a small bag with containers of fat-free dressing and fat-free sour cream.)

Use the substitution method again.

Instead of thick, fatty dressings, choose oil and vinegar or a vinaigrette, or even lemon. Enjoy the crunch and texture of the salad.

Instead of potatoes au gratin or buttery rice pilaf, ask for a plain baked potato. Squeeze lemon on it. Or ask for some low-fat milk and whip the milk into the insides of the potato. Or pour salsa on your spud for a spicy, fat-free treat. Bring along nonfat sour cream. Or use chili as a topping. (For instance, at Wendy's, order a plain baked potato and a side of their low-fat chili to put on it.) Better yet, ask for the restaurant's vegetables of the day, lightly steamed, in place of the potato.

Instead of red meat, choose grilled fish or chicken.

Instead of enchiladas and tamales at Mexican cantinas, order fajitas with lots of veggies. Eat with steamed corn tortillas. Or a light, fresh tostada with crisp leafy greens is a good pick. Skip the refried beans and rice or take them home for the kids. Enjoy the salsa without the chips. Take along some slices of jicama, celery, carrots, zucchini, and bell pepper for dipping. Ask for your own cup of chunky salsa and eat it, scoop by scoop, with a single chip.

Instead of eating "the whole enchilada," ask for a carry-out container when ordering and take half of your meal home for the next day's lunch.

Instead of ordering one entree per person, split an entree between the two of you. Then each of you fill up on a salad. You'll save money along with calories!

Instead of fried and sweet-and-sour Asian foods, choose those that are steamed and stir-fried.

Instead of ice cream, choose sherbet or nonfat, sugar-free frozen yogurt.

Have It Your Way

Burger King had a slogan for its fast-food establishment: Have it your way. Flame-broiled with pickle and tomato. Plain, no mayo. All beef, no bun. No beef, all bun. Whatever. It was your choice. That's unusual at a restaurant. Usually your waitress will tell you, "We can't make any substitutions." That's bad for a dieter. Almost all restaurant dishes are loaded with fats, sugars, starches, too much food, and too many calories. When eating healthy, there's no place like home. And here are some substitutes that will peel off those pounds:

Mayonnaise, dressings, dairy products: Low-fat instead of full fat

Mashed potatoes: Chicken broth and roasted garlic (clove or powder) instead of milk and butter

Toast, waffles, pancakes: Whole fruit preserves (no sugar added) instead of butter and syrup

Home-baked goodies: Prune puree instead of shortening and some of the sugar

Mochas and lattes: Canned nonfat milk instead of cream

Main dishes (casseroles, tacos, pizza, etc.): Chicken instead of red meat; ground turkey or soy instead of ground beef; plain yogurt instead of sour cream

Protein: Fish instead of any other meat (Dieters who ate fish twice a week lost twice as much weight!)

Sweets: Fruit instead of candy (Treat yourself to an exotic fruit frequently. Fresh pineapple is as sweet as any dessert!)

Try these tasty low fat recipes and tried-and-true dieter's tricks. Losing weight in a healthy, balanced way is a natural by-product of this plan. You really can have it your weigh!

6

"I Told You I Was Sick!"

This chapter originally had two other title options. The first was "Common Complaints of Women." Not very catchy (that's why we changed it!), but it got the point across. As we have traveled across America sharing the principles in *The Beautiful Balance* and *The Healthy Balance,* we have noticed common threads emerging in the tapestry of American women's lives. Just as there are certain temptations that are "common to man," there are certain illnesses that females often acquire and suffer. Many disorders develop thanks to our feminine anatomy and unique physical makeup. Our second title idea was "Misery Loves Company," but we ditched that because it sounded so negative. Isn't it true, though? It's a universal emotion. When we are suffering, we want to know we're not the only one suffering "just like this." Ever felt this way? Trust us, you are not alone in your misery!

One thing that I (Cynthia) have learned through my suffering is compassion for others. I remember thinking as I lay on the couch day after day, struggling with pain, "If I ever get well, I will listen to every sick person's story and show them mercy." It's been a blessing to be able to do that over the years—each one who has come to me for help and counsel is so precious. That brings us to our third secret in

---

Healthy Balance secret #3: Care for others like you care for yourself.

---

the *Healthy Balance* plan: *Care for others like you care for yourself.*

Nothing can heal you faster and sustain your health like taking your focus off yourself and reaching out to other people. The Bible teaches in Philippians 2:3–11:

> Do nothing from selfishness or empty conceit, but with humility of mind regard one another as more important than yourselves; do not merely look out for your own personal interests, but also for the interests of others. Have this attitude in yourselves which was also in Christ Jesus, who, although He existed in the form of God, did not regard equality with God a thing to be grasped, but emptied Himself, taking the form of a bond-servant, and being made in the likeness of men. Being found in appearance as a man, He humbled Himself by becoming obedient to the point of death, even death on a cross. For this reason also, God highly exalted Him, and bestowed on Him the name which is above every name, so that at the name of Jesus every knee will bow . . . and that every tongue will confess that Jesus Christ is Lord.

Healthy relationships with those around us provide us with the emotional state to truly heal any illness. We need the support of people to be whole, and they need that same encouragement. We were created to live in community and to thrive on giving to and receiving from others.

But Why This Title?

We decided on the title "I Told You I Was Sick!" after hearing a funny story by Dr. James Dobson. It seems that his mother always had various physical complaints, but nobody would listen to her. No one would take her ailments seriously. She asked to have the epitaph on her tombstone read, "I told you I was sick!" We laugh, but isn't it actually quite sad that sometimes it even takes death before our significant others believe we're honestly sick? Well, we believe you. Some of us have been there. We want to hear your stories. See if you recognize yourself in any of the complaints below.

Candida Control for Body and Soul

Do you feel sick all over, but doctors can't diagnose your problem? Are brain and neurological symptoms like spaciness, memory loss, headaches, and depression driving you crazy (literally, it seems)? Do you suffer from vaginal or bladder infections? Are certain foods, perfumes, and chemicals bothering you lately? Do you have intestinal complaints like constipation, diarrhea, abdominal pain, bloating, gas, or rectal itching? Does your period bring on symptoms of PMS, sugar cravings, fatigue, and other difficulties? Have you been on repeated rounds of antibiotics, Prednisone, and other steroids? Have you been pregnant multiple times, or have you taken the Pill for several years?

If you answered "yes" to some of these questions, there's a good chance that you too have a *Candida albicans* infection. A severe case of candida overgrowth, combined with my (Cynthia's) inherited low immunity and autoimmune problems, caused my varied symptoms. *Candida albicans* are microscopic, parasitic fungi that live in the warm, moist places of the human body: the digestive tract from mouth to rectum, the vagina, and other mucus membranes. These yeast organisms live quietly in the normal, healthy body, not causing a stir. But when conditions are right for them, they grow out of control, "colonizing," and taking over the system. According to microbiologists, if given the necessary food—sugar—fungus is the fastest-growing organism on earth.

As candida multiply and live out their life cycle of reproduction and death, they release forty different toxins into the bloodstream of their host. These toxins contribute to headaches and brain symptoms, muscle and joint pains, weakness, fatigue, the breakdown of the immune system, and other ailments. The sore throat, bowel symptoms, sinusitis, vaginitis, and bladder infections are localized irritations from colonized yeast. Swollen glands and low-grade afternoon fevers are the body's attempt to fight the infection. Because I have a genetic disposition to autoimmune illness, yeast overgrowth also throws me into a "lupuslike" flare complete with inflammation.

As the yeast continues to grow in the body, they burrow into the layers of the intestines, inflaming them and causing microscopic holes. These tiny openings allow undigested food particles into the bloodstream. This, combined with a patient's predisposition to an overactive immune system, can cause allergic reactions to foods and other substances.

You Gotta Have Hope!

This condition can seem hopeless. I know—I've lived with it for years. But rejoice! Like me, you can win the fight against candidiasis. You have to battle the little buggers on several fronts, however:

You kill them off (using prescription antifungals or natural treatments available at health stores).

You crowd them out. (In every intestinal tract grows many organisms, good and bad. The good bacteria, acidophilus, bifidus, and others, fight off yeast and other parasites.)

You starve them. (Eat only foods recommended here and in chapter 3.)

You fight them. (Strengthening your immune system to do battle is one of the wisest moves you can make not only for candidiasis, but for most other diseases too; read the section on immune dysfunction below.)

Let's take these steps for candida control one by one.

1. Kill them off.

If you have a severe yeast infection with multiple, miserable symptoms, you need relief fast! Diet and lifestyle changes, although very effective and highly recommended, take time. Fortunately, there are medications available to kill the yeast on contact. I took antifungal medications for eleven months under a doctor's watchful eye (testing me every month for liver abnormalities that can rarely occur with these medications). To rid myself of severe candida overgrowth, I had to occasionally go back on prescription medications. The newest drugs are Diflucan (fluconazole), Sporanox (itraconazole), Nizoral (ketoconazole), Vfend (voriconazole), and Amphotericin B (fungizone). These medications are powerful candida killers. They go into your bloodstream and destroy the fungi where they live and reproduce throughout the body. They should be used under a physician's supervision, preferably a preventative health doctor (they usually have a better understanding of this condition), and discontinued as soon as the condition is cleared. Nystatin (in tablet or oral powder form) kills candida in the mouth and digestive tract where most of the yeast colonize. Nystatin oral powder can also be diluted and used as a vaginal douche for vaginitis caused by candida. You can safely use Nystatin for longer periods of time than the more potent drugs. It is a very safe medication, even used on day-old newborns with oral thrush (also caused by candida).

The above yeast killers require a prescription by a medical doctor. If you prefer a more natural and inexpensive route, other remedies do work. Raw garlic is used in other countries as an effective antibiotic. Garlic also kills off yeasts and parasites. You can take it as the Russians do . . . raw. Crush a clove of garlic, put it on the back of the tongue, and swoosh it down with water. Eat some food immediately. This method helps eliminate *some* of the residual odor! Unfortunately, this method may cause you to lose more than parasites. Friends may abandon you too!

Deodorized garlic is available in pill form at health stores as aged garlic extract (Kyolic is a recommended brand). One good thing about garlic is that it builds up the immune system. One bad thing is that raw garlic also kills off good bacteria needed in your intestinal tract. Be sure to take probiotics (explained in the next few paragraphs) two hours after each "garlic gulp." Other products used by natural healers include taheebo tea (also called Pau D'Arco), grapefruit seed extract (sold as Citricidal), and caprylic acid (derived from coconut oil, the brand of caprylic acid recommended is Micopryl 680). These products are available from health food stores or can be ordered.

2. Crowd them out.

Who wants to live in a tiny, crowded compartment? We don't. You don't. And fortunately, yeast don't! Our bodies normally have good bacteria colonized in our intestines and vaginas. They keep candida and other microbes in check. But repeated antibiotic use and other factors like S.A.D.—the standard American diet—destroy the good bacteria in addition to the bad. The yeast are then allowed to proliferate.

It's important to kill off excess candida. But equally important is filling the body back up with good bacteria. There are 100 trillion microorganisms living in your intestinal tract. According to Elson Haas, M.D., author of *The Detox Diet,* there are more bacteria in a gram of human waste than there are stars in the known universe.[1]

Mind-boggling, isn't it? In a healthy body, the majority of microbes are good bacteria, or lactobacilli. This majority is what helps you have the healthy balance you need.

Lactobacilli, also called friendly flora or probiotics, are essential for your health. Here are some of the things that probiotics (*pro* means for, *biotics* means life) do for you:

Help lower your cholesterol.

Fight cancer.

Ward off stomach ulcers.

Protect against food poisoning.

Boost immune function.

Control growth of harmful microorganisms.

Contribute their antibacterial, antiviral, antifungal properties.

Prevent bowel problems like constipation, diarrhea, colitis, and irritable bowel.

Aid urinary tract infections.

Alleviate vaginitis.

Participate in the digestive process.

Manufacture some important B vitamins.

Produce digestive enzymes (including those to absorb calcium).

Maximize absorption and utilization of nutrients.

Provide vitamins, antioxidants, and cellular building blocks.

Guard against toxic body conditions.

Keep the colon clean with the proper acid balance.

Work against migraine headaches, rheumatic and arthritic complaints, and some skin conditions (acne, psoriasis, eczema).

This is just a partial list. Researchers are continually discovering new reasons to praise probiotics. You received your good bacteria as a gift from your mother, first from her own body when you were born, and then from her milk if you were breast-fed. If you were fed a healthy, lactobacilli-loving diet of fruits, vegetables, whole grains, legumes, low-fat yogurt, and pure water all of your life, you'd never have to supplement your good bacteria population.

But the average American diet, high in fat, meat, refined foods, caffeinated drinks, and the like, destroys lactobacilli, or at the very least is not conducive to its growth. Then we wipe out their numbers with broad-spectrum antibiotics (these drugs don't discriminate between good and bad "bugs"), and our defense system is further weakened. If we don't repopulate good intestinal flora, the harmful microbes that we ingest every day through food, water, and air take over and cause disease.

There are many different types of lactobacilli, but we'll just mention three. You have surely heard of the first, *Lactobacillus acidophilus,* or *L. acidophilus.* Many commercial yogurt brands claim to include this probiotic in their yogurts. This is an important probiotic. It lives in your small intestines, colonizing along the walls and forming your first line of defense against harmful invaders like *E. coli,* which can make you sick. In addition to protecting the mucosal lining of your small intestines, *L. acidophilus* heals, correcting the "leaky gut syndrome." It also produces hydrogen peroxide, acids, and natural antibiotics that create an environment hostile to pathogens.

Lactobacillus bifidus, or *L. bifidus,* live mostly in the large intestine and in small amounts in the lower small intestine. The colon retains the waste of the body, but if large amounts of bifidus are present, there is little putrefaction. Wastes are eliminated quickly. This allows no time for bad bacteria and yeasts to colonize or for carcinogenic agents to begin mutating cells. Bifidobacteria produce acetic and lactic acids, creating an unpleasant atmosphere for "bad bugs." Do you like to hang around in an unpleasant situation? Neither do they. When they holler, "We're outa here!" your health is protected. *L. bifidus* make their own B-complex vitamins and assist in other dietary processes.

Healthy Balance secret #4: Supplement daily with probiotics.

Another lactobacilli organism called *L. bulgaricus* is a transient bacteria that helps acidophilus and bifidus do their jobs. It's *L. bulgaricus* that cultures yogurt. As this bacteria grows in the milk, it transforms the liquid into a totally different substance with many unique health-giving properties. *L bulgaricus* also aids digestion and assimilation of nutrients.

Cynthia Shares

I can vouch for probiotic supplementation. You need two legs to stand on. I needed two things to get well. One was the *Healthy Balance* nutrition plan (without fruit, dairy, and high carbs for several years because of my candida problem). The other was the addition of probiotics into my diet. My health has been transformed for life! I've never felt better! I still take one probiotic capsule daily; when I'm ill, I take up to three. And of course, I encourage Charity and the rest of my family to supplement with probiotics too, especially when they are experiencing health problems or have taken a course of antibiotics.

After my health improved with the *Healthy Balance* plan, people came to me asking for help with their illnesses. I immediately put them on the program, with probiotic supplementation. It was amazing! They got well too, healing from conditions as varied as allergies and asthma to irritable bowel disease to immune dysfunctions.

Research is continually progressing in the field of microbiology, and specifically probiotic supplementation. Companies producing probiotic supplements must be committed to excellence, ethics, and correct manufacturing suggestions. For supplement companies that you can trust, please visit the following websites: www.lifebalanceladies.com or www.cynthiaculpallen .com. Or write for information:

Cynthia Culp Allen
1700 Airport Boulevard
Red Bluff, CA 96080

We want to help you get well!

How can you put these life-giving organisms back into your body? Our fourth secret in the *Healthy Balance* plan is: *Supplement daily with probiotics.*

Unfortunately all lactobacilli supplements are not created equal. Many commercial brands that you buy at health food stores offer nothing more than dead products. You may as well

Charity Chats

Let's face it: When Mom talks (whether we like what she's saying or not), we can't help but listen! And when my mom began experiencing huge improvements in her health after using probiotics, she began talking, and I got quite an earful, let me tell you! But like we often do with our mothers, I shrugged her off, saying that probiotics were great for her but not for me. After all, I was healthy—what need did I have for probiotic supplementation?

But I was knocked off my healthy high horse a few winters back, when I had just graduated college and was living on my own in the big city of Los Angeles without any medical insurance. For two months I had gone from one bout of the flu to the next and couldn't seem to shake it. In my desperation, I turned to "Dr. Mom." She reminded me of her success with probiotics and assured me that they could help strengthen my immune system as they had hers. I was looking for answers and agreed to give probiotics a try.

In about two weeks I was back to life as normal, full of energy, and a complete believer in probiotics. And guess what? Now it was me who began talking! Most of all I began talking to my athletic, health-conscious fiancé, Kelvin (who is now my husband), telling him all the ways probiotics had strengthened my mother's and my health and improved our lives. He said, "Probiotics, huh? They sound more like 'superman pills' to me!" But soon I was the one smiling when my big, tough guy sheepishly asked if he could try one of my "superman pills" one evening while eating dinner at my place!

Two years later, regular exercise, a balanced diet loaded with lots of fruits and vegetables, and daily "superman pill"-popping is the way of life in the Winters household. Kelvin and I look forward to passing these life-giving principles on to our future children, just as they were passed on in wisdom to us! What a valuable legacy—thanks, Dr. Mom!

throw your money out into the street rather than spend it on those brands! Lactobacilli are living organisms. They must be manufactured and handled a certain way to remain viable.

They must always be refrigerated but never frozen or over-heated. They come in different strains, almost like family lines, some more powerful and desirable than others. The products should remain in their natural environment, the supernatant (the culturing medium that they were made in, usually a milk/lactase base, but sometimes chickpea or garbanzo for dairy-free products). Here are supplemental suggestions:

Purchase probiotic capsules that provide at least 2 billion living bacteria through a guaranteed expiration date. They should be freeze-dried (lyophilization) and remain in the supernatant. You need to take separate powders or capsules of both acidophilus (DDS-1 super strain) and bifidus (Malyoth super strain).

It's important to eat a healthy diet that feeds the good bacteria. The *Healthy Balance* nutrition plan is perfect for this! Add natural yogurt to your diet. Yogurt is a predigested food because of the bacterial action of *L. bulgaricus.* Within an hour after eating a cup, 90 percent is digested. Milk, what yogurt is made from, is only 30 percent digested in an hour. Plus the calcium in the yogurt is absorbed better.

In 1908, Dr. Elie Metchnikoff, a Russian biologist who won the Nobel Prize for Physiology and Medicine, wrote *The Prolongation of Life* after observing various healthy societies of people who lived extended life spans. The key ingredient in each group was the inclusion of cultured foods like yogurt, kefir, cheese, sauerkraut, and soy products in their daily diets. Civilization has been ingesting cultured foods since man's early days, as far back as 9000 B.C. In recent years, Americans have rediscovered our ancestors' tonic. The dairy shelves of our stores are filled with brand after brand of cultured foods. Be sure you choose products that contain live cultures and few fillers. Learn to enjoy plain yogurt minus all the sugary fruit and fuss. Your friendly flora will love you for it!

First, try a cleansing regime to rid your body of accumulated toxins (for a variety of fun and beneficial cleansing programs, watch for our upcoming book in the LifeBalance series, *The Inner Balance*). Then begin taking effective probiotic supplements. It will change your life! You'll serve God with a stronger, healthier, more energetic body. Sound too good to be true? It can happen to you!

3. Starve them.

The smart army general doesn't keep feeding the enemy, making him stronger. If you want to win your battle against candida, you too must use the effective tool of deprivation. Yeast thrives on sugar of any kind. It makes no difference if it's natural or not—table sugar, honey, fruit, candy, cookies, cakes, pies, ice cream—all the things we love but don't thrive on! For a severely infected individual, even lactose (milk sugar) or too many carbohydrates may have to go for a while. Nutritionally deficient products made with flour, and even whole-grain products, are all converted to sugar in the bloodstream. To get well, you must eliminate all sugar and goodies made of sugar. Go as far as checking labels! Prepared foods in cans, bottles, and packages have sugar more often than not.

For a month, commit yourself to eat a whole foods diet as described in chapter 3, but minus the fruits and milk products (except 1 daily cup of plain yogurt with live cultures). You can enjoy protein choices like lean meats, poultry, eggs, fish, and soy. Also eat lots of fresh vegetables (excluding starchy vegetables like potatoes, sweet potatoes and yams, corn, beets). Add some good fats like olive oil, flaxseed oil, Balanced Butter, avocados, and nuts. Limited portions of legumes are acceptable. Although these are heavyweights in both protein and carbs, beans are hard for the yeast to break down to use as food. Finally, drink lots of pure water and herbal teas. There have been times in my life (Cynthia)—years actually—when all I've eaten are protein foods, vegetables (nothing starchy), and good fats. Period. I needed this strict diet to get well. Do not cheat—your health can't afford it! Continue on your antiyeast medications and probiotics.

When your symptoms disappear, you may add dairy products (nonfat if you need to lose weight) back into your diet. See how your body responds. Try adding a low-sugar fruit (apples, melons, or berries) and be aware of any returning symptoms. I still can't overeat fruit after eighteen years of candida control; I have a chronic condition. Keep a food journal. Record in your "New You" notebook the way your body responds to the foods you feed it. You'll begin to see what your individual needs are as far as avoiding certain foods or repeating them.

Do not add sugar and its products back into your life, however. These "treats" are detrimental to anyone's health, especially yours. After a few weeks on the *Healthy Balance* diet, you will lose your sugar craving. Sugar and her accomplices will lose their power over your life. You'll develop a longing for whole, natural, health-giving foods.

4. Fight them.

When you are in the middle of a severe candida infection, you know you're in a war. Many times it seems like a battle for your very life. One client said to me (Cynthia), "It feels like my body just might blow up!"

A healthy immune system fights candida for you. It's your best weapon against this infection and others. Read the next section to discover how you can develop an immune system that fights for you and not against you.

A warning: Be prepared for some die-off symptoms. Sometimes when an individual begins a candida control program, the complaints temporarily worsen. This is because the medications, diet, and probiotics are doing their jobs—killing off the yeast. This is a good thing! But when candida die, they release potent toxins into your bloodstream. These toxins cause symptoms like brain fog, headaches, muscle and joint pains, fatigue, and other symptoms. You feel like you have the flu! If needed, take a few sick days off work until these die-off symptoms stop (trust us, they really will go away when the candida count is down!). Pamper yourself with warm bubble baths and spa treatments (see our next book, *The Inner Balance*), two-hour naps, delicious, nutritious foods, a funny movie to laugh your cares away, a heart-to-heart on the phone with a friend, and a good book to distract you from your woes until they're gone for good.

Immune Dysfunction

Your immune system is the guardian of your health and well-being. When the immune system goes haywire, a person can suffer from myriad ailments running the gamut from frequent colds to cancer. Building strong immune performance is the most important function of the *Healthy Balance* plan, crucial to robust living. Most people are born with stable immune systems. Through the years, problems develop to burden the body: nutritional deficiencies due to poor diet, lack of exercise, exposure to chemicals, pollutants and allergens (like molds), food, inhalant, and chemical allergies, smoking and other detrimental habits, overuse of antibiotics, overgrowth of yeasts and other parasites, stress, and others.

When the system is overloaded, it begins to break down. In his book *Viral Immunity,* J. E. Williams, O.M.D., lists the stages of immune system compromise:

Level One: Frequent bouts with fatigue, headaches, aches and pains, recurrent colds and viruses, frequent allergies.

Level Two: The symptoms of level one increased in severity, longevity, and frequency. Constant fatigue. Sleep disturbances. Memory and thinking also affected.

Level Three: Infections from fungus and bacterial agents (*Candida albicans,* sinusitis), shingles and other herpes virus infections. Nervous system symptoms develop, causing unusual conditions (MS-like weakness in extremities, loss of balance, inflammation, numbness, tingling), severe memory and cognitive impairment, depression and anxiety disorders, unable to handle stress.

Level Four: At this stage, diseases develop (MS, CFIDS, AIDS). All symptoms of level one through level three worsen. Fatigue is disabling.

Level Five: Complete immune failure. Death from opportunistic infections and cancer.[2]

This sounds scary, we know. But the good news is that you can turn these stages around. We hope to catch you back at level one or two. But even the other stages can be reversed through the *Healthy Balance* plan. The root of the problem is an imbalanced lifestyle—a junk diet, no exercise, little time to rest and renew, stress at home or work, and neglect of one's spiritual life. Change these foundational factors and you change your life!

Crucial components to good immune function are:

Healthy diet and supplementation. Eat the ripe fruits and fresh vegetables, lean meats, grains and legumes, non-fat dairy, and healthy oils suggested in the *Healthy Balance* plan. But don't overeat, even on these good foods. When I (Cynthia) was so sick, if I ate healthy balanced meals in small portions, I improved. When I overate, even nutritiously, all my symptoms flared miserably, sending me to bed. The "systems overload" set me back several days until my body recovered from the assault. Eat wisely, in moderation. Take a multivitamin and mineral supplement to ensure daily requirements are met. Vitamins that are especially important for strong immunity are Vitamin A (the anti-infection vitamin; raises IGA levels, the antibodies that protect your mucus membranes, your immune system's first defense), Vitamin C (most important for immunity),Vitamin E (builds the body's defense), and zinc (a mineral that boosts the immune system's response).

If you suffer from food allergies, experiment with the Cavewoman Diet. For one week, eat only foods that you rarely eat. It could be anything from artichokes to turkey to lentils. Choose a handful of foods that seldom grace your dinner table and feast on those for one week. Eat all you want of whole foods (not packaged), avoiding the foods that are common allergens—eggs, milk, wheat, corn, tomatoes, chocolate, sugar, white potatoes, and so on, doing without your favorite foods. Many times our "comfort foods" are the very foods we build immunities against because we eat them too often. Note in your "New You" notebook whether your allergic symptoms diminish or disappear or if you have any reactions. After the week is up, add one other food back in each day, recording your body's response. This is one of the best ways to see what you're allergic to. Rotate the foods that you can tolerate so that you eat them only every fourth day. (You can keep track of your rotations in your "New You" notebook.) I (Cynthia) was so allergic at one time that I weighed a little over 100 pounds at 5'8". There were few foods I could eat. If I ate my trigger foods, they would send me to the hospital emergency room with anaphylaxis. The Cavewoman Diet helped me discover that I was severely allergic to wheat (it gave me my horrid brain symptoms described in chapter 2) and had severe sensitivities to sugar and fruit (the candida). I also reacted to dairy products, eggs, corn, and a few other foods. In time, my body healed because I adhered to the *Healthy Balance* program, rotated my foods for a year or so, took probiotics, and avoided my allergens. Now I can eat everything but sugar (rarely!).

Exercise. Natural killer cells that attack infection and other immune system fighters increase with exercise, as do levels of hormones specific for good immune function. In addition, physical activity regulates all the functions of the body, which in turn improves immunity. Ninety percent of Americans agree that exercise is a key factor in good health. But only 15 percent get the exercise they need. Over 76 percent neglect to do even one lively activity per week. Yet 75 percent of us will die of preventable diseases.[3] Get moving! Moderation in all things, however. Research also demonstrates that excessive, traumatic workouts tear down the immune system.

Sleep. The hours that you are asleep in bed are the restorative part of your day. Most individuals require eight hours of sleep; those suffering from infections of any kind need nine or ten. Lack of sleep causes vulnerability to viruses and bacteria and decreases the level of natural killer cells.

Pure water and air. Milk may do a body good. But, with apologies to the dairy industry, there is a beverage we need even more. Pure water. Drink plenty of it—eight glasses a day to keep lymph fluids moving, along with the other benefits that we discussed earlier. Studies have also shown that higher oxygen levels destroy bacteria, fungus, and viruses, so inhale completely when you exercise and practice deep breathing when you relax.

Diabetes

There are two types of diabetes mellitus: Type I, or juvenile diabetes, occurring mostly in children and young adults, and Type II, adult-onset diabetes. The disease is caused from a defect in insulin production by the pancreas. Insulin is needed by the body to utilize glucose for energy. Diabetes complications are the third leading cause of death in the United States. Diet affects this disease as much as it does candida. Overweight people who eat diets high in refined, processed foods and sugary goodies and low in fiber are more likely to develop diabetes as they grow older.

Barry Sears, Ph.D., in his book *Enter the Zone,* offers the theory that "food should be understood as a drug."[4] (Remember the theories of Hippocrates, the Chinese, and other ancients: food is medicine.) Sears outlines a nutritional program that, if followed, he claims will control your hormonal responses to food like a powerful drug. I (Cynthia) read several of Dr. Sears's books hoping to find help for my mother, who is suffering from complications of diabetes. It's a great plan, but so complex. The key components of the diet are to equalize food blocks of protein, carbohydrates, and fats into the perfect ratios. I was never good in math, so it was too much for me to figure out. If you have a technical mind, you might enjoy reading Sears's books. But you can hold to his basic ideas as you eat freely from the *Healthy Balance* plan. (A free spirit like me wants freedom within a guideline. I only stay on those rigid eating plans about one week max. What about you?) Diabetics should eat a protein portion and carb portion of the same size at each meal. Take a little fat with these foods too. Eating a wide variety of nonstarchy vegetables will fill you up without affecting insulin levels. You can enjoy salads with healthy salad dressings since fat is not the issue for you.

Fibromyalgia and Chronic Fatigue Syndrome

The achy-breaky condition called Fibromyalgia (FM) is diagnosed more frequently these days, with over 80 percent of patients being women. Most complain of body pain, muscle achiness, morning stiffness, sleep disturbances, and fatigue. Doctors press "tender points" on the body to confirm a diagnosis. Chronic fatigue immune deficiency syndrome (CFIDS) presents itself with sore throat, achiness, fatigue, headache, and cognitive dysfunction. Like many of these modern-day epidemics, the cause is unknown. Having suffered with these conditions myself (Cynthia), I believe that these disabling disorders originate from body conditions similar to those discussed in the first two sections in this chapter, candida and immune dysfunction.

In an article entitled, "Yeast and the CFIDS Patient," Dr. Jorge Flechas wrote:

> In our CFIDS population we found an overgrowth of Candida Albicans on the mucous tissues of the body to be a common occurrence.... Based on the work in our office we hypothesize that the T-cell defects of CFIDS allow Candida Albicans to grow.... It is important that an aggressive antiyeast program be in place for the CFIDS patient until his/her immune system returns to its normal state.[5]

Follow the diet we suggest in the candida control section. Practice the principles of the *Healthy Balance* lifestyle and see if your symptoms diminish. Chart your body's response in your "New You" notebook. Fibromyalgia patients should begin mild walking immediately. Studies have shown that moderate exercise alleviates much of the achiness, joint stiffness, and depression associated with the condition. As soon as CFIDS sufferers gain some strength, they should begin to exercise, a step at a time. When I (Cynthia) began my recovery plan, I could only walk several steps before lying down again. But I added to my daily exercise little by little, until I was finally walking two hours a day, and even jogging. I began feeling fantastic, better than ever before. Lack of exercise creates lack of energy. The longer you stay in bed, the weaker you become. When the diet does its magic, get up and get moving for your health's sake.

Female Difficulties

Premenstrual syndrome, or PMS, is that week in the month, near that time of month, when you nearly want to kill someone. One minute you're yelling at the kids, the next you're crying over something your husband said. The neighbors drive you nuts, and you've given up on your best girlfriend. Things look mighty bleak, and there's no light at the end of the tunnel. It's a wild and crazy time in a woman's life.

One time an old man paying for groceries at a country store leaned over to me (Cynthia) as I was standing next to him in line.

"Wanna hear a good joke?" the old farmer asked, stuffing his change back into the pocket of his red flannel shirt.

"Sure! Why not?" I answered. I love a good joke.

He launched into it. "Why do they call it PMS?"

I shrugged.

"Because Mad Cow Disease was already taken!" He hooted and hollered all the way out of the store.

"Male chauvinist," I said under my breath, glaring after him.

But we have to laugh at the clever joke. PMS symptoms drive us (and our families) straight up the proverbial wall. Some of the complaints that women report are nervous tension, anxiety, irritability, water retention, bloating, weight gain, craving for sweets, increased appetite, palpitations, fatigue, fainting spells, "the shakes," headaches and brain symptoms like depression, withdrawal, insomnia, forgetfulness, confusion, and sometimes even suicidal feelings. When I suffered with it, there were times when I felt like a crazy old cow! But good news: After clearing myself of candida and adhering to the *Healthy Balance* diet, I've never had PMS again. Charity never suffered from PMS because she has eaten healthy balanced meals since she was young. Before her period, she just cuts back on sugar and fruit in her diet. And of course, probiotic supplementation helps too.

Hormonal changes involved in the menstrual cycle encourage candida growth. The normal American diet feeds the increased candida, which heightens symptoms. It's a vicious cycle: more yeast, more cravings for sweets to feed the yeast, more sugary foods, the yeast proliferate, more symptoms . . .

Many doctors agree with this theory that yeast overgrowth contributes to PMS. In an article in *Redbook* magazine, Dr. Pamela Morford, a Tucson, Arizona, gynecologist, reported that "the premenstrual problems of at least 90 percent of my patients can be traced back to chronic candidiasis. I've found that when I give these patients anticandida therapy, they get better."[6]

In PMS, as in other diseases and disorders, there are many factors that figure into the causes of the condition. But try the candida control program for a month or two, and evaluate your body's response. Ask your family if they notice a difference. Trust us, those you live with will be the first to help you stay on your program if it helps you feel better.

Unlike these other conditions, menopause is a natural occurrence in a woman's life. "The change," as it is often called, transpires when a female stops ovulating and menstruating. Hormone levels greatly decrease during this time. Some women experience symptoms like fatigue, hot flashes, night sweats, mood swings, dizziness, anxiety and depression, low sex drive, dry skin, incontinence, and insomnia. Low estrogen levels also contribute to osteoporosis, or brittle bones.

The diet, exercise, and lifestyle suggestions in *The Healthy Balance* will greatly diminish any unpleasant side effects of menopause, as will control of emotions. This is a transition time in life, a change that takes from one to five years. Some women go through it symptom-free. But for those who suffer, here are a few additions to the *Healthy Balance* program.

East Meets West

Japanese women don't suffer through menopause like American women do. A report in *Lancet* (the British medical journal) explains that women in Japan eat more phytoestrogens (or plant estrogens). Foods like soybeans and soy products, tofu, miso, dates, pomegranites, and flaxseeds are rich in these composites. Although not the actual hormone, these plant substances act like estrogen in the body, alleviating menopausal symptoms. In addition, a nutrient from rice bran (gamma-oryzanol) reduces women's postmenopausal complaints. The mainstay of the Japanese diet is rice. Ginseng, gotu kola, and dong quai are herbs used to aid in estrogen production and relieve symptoms like hot flashes, vaginal dryness, and depression. Several teas have been shown to be strengthening and calming during this time, including green tea, licorice, chamomile, and kombucha.

Osteoporosis

Porous bones become a problem for many women when their estrogen production declines. Postmenopausal women should get 1500–2000 mg of calcium a day through foods like nonfat dairy products, leafy greens, almonds, salmon, and supplementation. Weight-bearing exercises like walking, jogging, and step aerobics help build and maintain bone mass, as does weight lifting. Sodas and other carbonated beverages should be kept to a minimum or eliminated. Studies show that the phosphates in these popular drinks cause the body to expel calcium along with the phosphates. Caffeine also depletes calcium levels, as do high-protein diets. Moderation (or even abstention, in some cases!) in all things.

High Blood Pressure

High blood pressure or hypertension has been called the "silent killer." Unlike the illnesses mentioned above, it develops with little or no symptoms. Thirty-five million Americans have high blood pressure, but only twenty million know it. When hypertension is advanced, it can cause headaches, rapid pulse, shortness of breath, dizziness, and vision problems. More women than men die of the complications of high blood pressure, which include kidney failure, heart failure, and stroke. That's the bad news.

The good news is that high blood pressure is preventable. Key to maintaining normal blood pressure is getting to, and staying at, your desired weight. Stick with the *Healthy Balance* plan (naturally high in fiber) until you are slim and energetic. A salt-free diet is helpful in lowering pressure. If "salt-free" is synonymous with "gag-me," try some of the herbal salt replacements like Herbamare or Bragg's Amino Acids for flavor.

Another important lifestyle change is to add mild to moderate exercise to your day. Check with your physician, and then begin a walking program. Not only will the exercise "lower your blood pressure" physiologically, but psychologically as well. Exercise is a known stress reducer.

Supplements that are useful in controlling hypertension include garlic (try Kyolic Aged Garlic capsules, which are minus the odor, by Wakunaga); calcium (1500 mg–3000 mg), magnesium (750–1000 mg) and potassium (see product label, or eat a banana a day); and essential fatty acids available in flax oil, olive oil, and evening primrose oil. Herbs that help control blood pressure are chamomile, fennel, hawthorn berries, parsley, rosemary, and cayenne (capsicum). Begin herbal supplementation slowly until you see what your body will tolerate.

The Cancer Answer for Body and Soul

One of the most grim pronouncements a patient can hear from a doctor is, "I'm sorry, but you have cancer." This dreaded disease is prevalent in our society. Check out these statistics: Cancer causes one in five of all deaths. It strikes three of four American families. Over 1.9 million new cases of cancer will be diagnosed this year.[7] Every forty-five seconds a U.S. citizen dies of the disease—that's 1900 Americans each day.[8] This illness will affect one in three people alive today. Is there an answer for this epidemic? You can decide for yourself after careful consideration of the facts.

To find the answer, we must first ask more questions. What causes cancer? At this point no one knows for sure. But more and more, evidence is pointing to environmental agents that cause cell abnormalities, cells that are not strong enough to withstand today's onslaught of carcinogens. Cause and effect figures into the equation. Smokers or people who work around asbestos frequently develop lung cancer. Sun worshipers reap skin damage and the accompanying malignancies. Alcohol abusers are diagnosed more often with mouth, throat, and liver cancers. There is now confirmation that a high-fat, low-fiber diet is influential in the development of colon, breast, prostate, and other cancers. Some researchers fear that dietary influence is even greater. According to Roy Walford, M.D., author of *Beyond the 120 Year Diet,* up to 90 percent of cancers develop due to environmental factors, with diet being the most important factor.[9]

How can nutrition play such an important role in the anticancer fight? Is the typical American diet to blame for many of the life-threatening conditions of the nation's population?

Cancer begins when cells duplicate themselves uncontrollably. Cell reproduction is not an abnormal occurrence in the body. Our bodies were ingeniously programmed to create more cells for the healing of injuries. You've observed new skin growing over a cut on your hand. When healing is complete, the cell reproduction stops.

Not so in cancer cells. Something causes the reproduction mechanism to go crazy, out of control. Cells reproduce, and if unchecked, continue to grow, creating tumors (or excessive white counts in malignancies of the blood). These cancerous cells can metastasize (spread) to other parts of the body where they continue their uncontrolled growth. When this abnormal overgrowth interferes with the body's ability to function properly, illness or death result.

Many scientists believe that free radical damage is the major factor in cancer. Free radicals are atoms containing one unpaired electron. Another atom or molecule can then pair with this atom, creating a chemical reaction that causes damage (sometimes irreversible) at the cell level. Damage too many cells and you get sick. The normal body incurs some free radicals on a small scale. For instance, free radicals are released during digestion and assimilation of food. But a healthy, normal body neutralizes any damage done. Excessive free radicals damage cells to the point of illness. A diet high in fat creates more free radicals. Even worse is the practice of cooking fats at high temperatures (think of all the fried fast foods our culture consumes!).

Recent studies and subsequent writings confirm these theories. The *Journal of the American Cancer Institute* reported that women who eat more than 10 grams of saturated fats a day have a 20 percent greater risk of developing ovarian cancer.[10] There are 8 grams of fat in a muffin alone, 31 grams in a Big Mac! Do yourself a favor—pack a brown-bag lunch of fresh fruits and wholesome, low-fat foods!

More and more, research is pointing toward fresh fruits and vegetables as the answer for cancer. It's been called "produce prevention." Studies have found that common cancers are reduced by 50 percent in countries where about a pound of fruits and vegetables are eaten a day. Also, in several studies done by C. H. Barrows, Jr., and G. C. Kokkonen (recorded in *Nutritional Approach to Aging Research*), the incidence of breast cancer was knocked down to zero by eating a high-nutrition, low-cal diet like the one recommended in *The Healthy Balance*.[11] Cancer specialist Mitchell Gaynor, M.D., stated in a *Newsweek* article that "eating the right foods is as specific to stopping cancer before it starts as wearing a seat belt is to lowering your risk of a fatal automobile accident."[12]

The proper diet negates free radicals and strengthens the body. This eating program must be full of antioxidants, a group of vitamins, minerals, and enzymes that protect the body and heal it of free radical damage. Here are some of the common antioxidants and the foods they are in (available at supermarkets and health food stores, all can also be purchased as supplements in addition to food):

Alpha-lipoic acid, in most fruits and vegetables

Coenzyme Q10, also in all fresh foods

Cysteine, a sulfur-bearing amino acid in garlic, onions, and cruciferous veggies

Ginkgo Biloba (from the ginkgo tree), buy supplements

Glutathione, an enzyme produced by your body, made from cysteine and other amino acids; take n-acetyl-cysteine supplements for more glutathione

Grape seed extract, a flavenoid found in purple and green fruits (especially grapes) and veggies, or supplement

Green tea, buy bagged or loose tea leaves (Epigallo catechin gallate ester is the most powerful antioxidant that green tea is known for. Buy the finer green teas!)

Melatonin, a hormone that the pineal gland produces in response to the presence or absence of light. (Get at least fifteen minutes of sunshine a day! It will lift your mood and help you sleep.)

Pycnogenol, pine bark extract in supplements

Selenium, in wheat germ, bran, tuna, onions, tomatoes, broccoli. Also supplements. The *Journal of the American Medical Association* reported a 50 percent reduction in cancer deaths among diagnosed patients who took 100 mcg of selenium twice a day (this mineral can be toxic—55 to 65 mcg a day is advisable).

Superoxide Dismutase, in barley grass, broccoli, brussels sprouts, cabbage, wheatgrass, and most green plants

Vitamin A and Beta-carotene, in liver, carrots and yellow or orange fruits and vegetables, eggs, milk, and dairy products

Vitamin C, in citrus fruits, berries, green and leafy vegetables, tomatoes, cauliflower, potatoes, sweet potatoes

Vitamin E, in wheat germ, soybeans, vegetable oils, broccoli, brussels sprouts, leafy greens, spinach, whole-grain cereals, eggs

Zinc, in meats like beef, lamb, and pork, wheat germ, brewer's yeast, pumpkin seeds, eggs, nonfat dry milk, ground mustard

Research confirms that fruits and vegetables are most important in preventing and fighting cancer. Doesn't this take us right back to the beginning and God's instructions for the human's diet? We have wandered so far from the Garden. There, in that place and time, God programmed our bodies to want and need live, fresh produce. We still desire those foods today, but we try to satisfy the God-given desire with dry, stale, packaged, and processed fillers. Our bodies are protesting!

The battle has begun. Cancer is fought on two levels. One: Furnish your body with what it needs to fight free radical damage, as discussed above. Two: Build up your immune system to battle the disease (see the immune dysfunction section on page 151). Even healthy folks have cancer cells circulating in their bodies. But a robust individual's powerful immune system destroys the cancer cells before they can accumulate and harm normal tissue.

To prevent cancer or heal yourself of the disease, the *Healthy Balance* lifestyle offers an answer to consider. It will empty your body of toxins and build up your immune system

Cynthia Shares

In 1994, I had seven doctors "diagnose" me with metastasized ovarian cancer. I remember those two weeks before surgery. Although I trusted Christ for my eternity, what about my here-and-now with five children still at home? Such a hopeless feeling! And the medical profession offered me no encouragement. But we have confidence in God first of all. He is the Great Physician. The Lord has a compassionate "bedside manner," and he's the Healer of all our diseases.

Don't ever allow a doctor to tell you how long you have or how long a loved one has to live. Only the almighty God knows the number of our days. And with him, nothing (no situation) is impossible! In those two weeks before surgery, I researched and studied every method, conventional and unconventional, to fight cancer. My battle plan was firmly established before they ever wheeled me into the operating room. Mainly, I planned to survive!

Thankfully, the prayers of many were answered and doctors found no cancer in exploratory surgery. They removed my huge tumor (and my uterus and one ovary). After snooping around in there for a while, Sherlock Holmes–style, they stitched me back up. I'm still a medical mystery to those at the hospital who don't believe in miracles!

and organs to fight disease—any disease. In his wonderful book *Food as Medicine,* Dr. Dharma Khalsa writes: "Every major ailment has a specific natural food prescription that can reverse its course. This is the cutting edge of medicine."[13]

In your fight for good health, be sure to add these four elements to your life:

First, fresh fruits and vegetables, preferably organic. (Cancer patients don't need any more carcinogens.) Eat them as close to nature as possible—raw, juiced, in salads, lightly steamed. Your body must have the natural enzymes they provide in their natural state to digest, assimilate, and heal. The *Healthy Balance* diet as outlined in chapter 3 will work well for you, but add even more vegetables through juices and raw salads to boost your immune system.

Second, begin the diet with a three-day cleanse or longer. Our next book, *The Inner Balance,* features cleanses for every lifestyle. Do this cleanse once a month. The immune system destroys cancer cells during a cleanse or fast. Stay on the internal balance program.

Third, add exercise to the *Healthy Balance* plan of good nutrition. Occasional cleansing, walking, and resting will allow your body to heal itself. Your body was created to respond to a balanced lifestyle. When you give it God's best, your body will reward you with life.

Fourth, add one more thing to your anticancer program: hope. This is the next secret, number five, in the *Healthy Balance* plan: *Add hope to your life.* Hope for this life through the healing power of your Creator God, and hope for the life to come through the saving grace of Jesus Christ.

Healthy Balance secret #5: Add hope to your life.

We can also find hope in those who have gone before us. Many patients have healed themselves of end-stage cancers when medical doctors had given them up for dead. Eileen Gray, a friend of Cynthia, is living proof of a homemade cancer miracle. Years ago, after her lymphoma diagnosis, she educated herself on nutrition. Eileen took the *Healthy Balance* plan to the extreme, eating only raw plant foods. And her health is better today than it was before her cancer diagnosis. She now has hope that she will live to raise her three beautiful children adopted from Vietnam.

Remember Jesus' words: Ask, seek, knock, and it will be given, found, and opened up to you. Courageous (and cured) people questioned, researched, sought out, discovered, devised a plan, and disciplined themselves to that plan. And they won! They beat the battle of cancer, our number two killer—and you can too!

The Deadliest Cancer

There is a disease that is more dangerous than cancer of the body. It's cancer of the soul. Sin is the cancer that eats away at the heart of us—the part of us that's made in "the image of God." All evil is a curse. But the pervasive sin we're considering here is bitterness. Cancer kills by taking over the body. Bitterness does the same thing, taking over the body of Christ.

> See to it that no one comes short of the grace of God; that no root of bitterness springing up causes trouble, and by it many be defiled.
>
> Hebrews 12:15

Most of us, when we are bitter, don't keep it to ourselves, do we? Our negative thoughts and feelings become public knowledge as we spread them around, causing strife. A bit of gossip here, slander over there, whisper, whisper. . . . A sarcastic comment about the person who has hurt us, whether she knew what she was doing or not. We want to hurt that person like she has hurt us, right?

The Lord says vengeance is his. He will take care of the unrepentant offender. But remember, if they are repentant and they've confessed to God and asked your forgiveness,

Jesus took care of that transgression on the cross. It's dead and buried with him. Leave it there.

Can you forgive? Jesus says you can. He told Peter to forgive seventy times seven. That's 490 times, if you don't have a calculator. That's a lot. Of course, if the offender is your husband, parent, or child and you're living with them, the total offenses may max out above that number! But you get the point. Jesus was saying to keep on forgiving. Don't give up on graciousness. Don't come short of the grace of God. For by the measure that you forgive, he said, you shall be forgiven. That's the part that always bites, doesn't it?

We certainly want to be forgiven. Don't you? The Bible assures us that all of the sins we've sought forgiveness for and repented of, our Lord has graciously forgiven. That is how we can forgive others. On our knees. In gratitude and dependence. Through our own admittance of sin and confession of it. Through prayer, asking Christ to forgive others through us. Allowing his love to flood our hearts and lives. Forgiveness is freeing. It's good for your health. And it's commanded.

> Let all bitterness and wrath and anger and clamor and slander be put away from you, along with all malice. Be kind to one another, tender-hearted, forgiving each other, just as God in Christ also has forgiven you.
>
> Ephesians 4:31–32

Those slanderers with a root of bitterness are like free radicals in the body of Christ. They go around doing damage and starting emotional fires here and there, until the fellowship goes up in smoke. Over and over, Scripture tells us to avoid people like these. Do whatever it takes to stay away from them. I (Cynthia) have had to step away from certain friendships because they tempted me to gossip and slander people (and of course, I was probably a temptation to some myself!). I want to obey the Lord. My desire is to become like Jesus Christ. Both Charity and I want to become beautiful, healthy, balanced women of God, both in body and soul.

The *Beautiful Balance* and the *Healthy Balance* programs are for the total you. The *Life Balance* plan is a satisfying and fruitful way to live. But it does take some decision, action, restraint, and denial of desires. These choices involve long-lived health and beauty. They have eternal consequences and are not just for "instant gratification." Disciplining our lives in this way is a small price to pay to reap huge rewards that last for eternity.

> Doctors diagnose, food cures, and God heals.
>
> yoga nutritional therapist Yogi Bhajan

7

Feel-Good Fitness
for the Total You

Don't you wish you could take your body into a body shop, like your husband does the car, and get a complete overhaul? Just a simple, annual appointment, and you're good to go. No pain for the gain. No sweatin' to the oldies. We could eat whatever we wanted and still fit in our clothes beautifully.

Life would be so pleasant if that were possible, right?

Wrong!

If that were society's method of staying fit, we'd all miss out on one of our greatest blessings: *the joy of movement*. God created humans to be movers and shakers. Our bodies were made to move and to enjoy the activity. Just like we talk ourselves *into* overeating as adults, we talk ourselves *out of* action.

Watch your children or a park full of kids at play. Do you see one of them sitting still? Okay, we may see the one who just got into trouble sulking over at the picnic table. Time-outs happen. But normal children want to move. They feel like they'll die if they're forced to sit still. We adults have to train ourselves to become slugs. We do it gradually, year after year. Your energy continued from high school into college, surely. Then you got married, and it was all downhill from there. So comfortable, enjoying life. Quiet evenings at home curled up on the couch watching TV. Or all those dinners out to celebrate "our two-month/three-month . . . anniversary," and so on. (Just ask me, Charity!) Making all those gourmet meals to impress the new hubby, keeping house, working at your job. No time for fitness. Then the kids came and you exhausted yourself chasing after them all day. Who needs exercise? All you wanted to do in your free time was flop on the couch and veg with Oprah, right?

> According to a study from the United Kingdom, people there burn about 800 calories less per day than they did in 1970.
>
> *Prevention—Women's Health Today*

Unfortunately, inactivity breeds inertia. *Inertia* is defined in dictionaries as the tendency of a body to resist acceleration; the tendency of a body at rest to remain at rest; resistance to motion, action, or change.

Couch potatoes have very slack metabolisms. In not moving, we lose muscle strength and energy. Without bodily movement, this process of burning foods for energy (metabolism) slows tremendously, using fewer and fewer calories. That means we must eat less and less but still gain more and more pounds. This is the reverse of what we want to happen! And if we don't make a mental change now, things will only worsen as we age. Researchers have pointed out that a lack of daily exercise is as detrimental to the body as smoking half a pack of cigarettes a day! Physically and spiritually, it's important *not* to do certain things. But just as important is the *To Do* list of the things you know are right and good: "To one who knows the right thing to do and does not do it, to him it is sin" (James 4:17).

We're not saying it's a sin not to exercise. But follow the point here: We know it's right to read our Bibles and pray.

These activities strengthen our souls and spirits. In the same way, we know that God made our bodies to need good nutrition and activity. Our carnal nature keeps us from doing the very things we know are good for us! (Check out the apostle Paul's confession in Romans 7.) In the power of the Holy Spirit, we can adapt new, fruitful habits for body and soul.

Body Basics

As we grow older, it's harder to keep our bodies in tip-top shape. It's a fact of life that youths don't need to do much to maintain fit bodies. Growth spurts rev up a teen's metabolism so she can eat more and still keep her slim figure. Girls are usually more active than adult females anyway. They burn more calories, use more muscles. Genetics has a lot to do with when a woman loses this advantage. Some females notice it in their twenties, some after childbirth, while others (for instance, many models) don't need to do anything into their forties, when time finally catches up with them. Metabolism slows down, as does activity level, and priorities change. (Ease and comfort begin to reign supreme!) Skin loses its elasticity, and of course, gravity takes its inevitable toll. The spread of middle age is upon us. The matronly image. But this chapter offers hope that we can maintain our figures and health well into advanced years through moderate exercise.

The Magic of Movement

Throughout this book we've given you secrets for healthy, balanced living for body and soul. Here we offer secret num-

Cynthia Shares

There was a time in my life when I could only walk a minute at a time, if that. I remember it so well. I was beginning the slow recovery from my illness (again!) and wanted to build up my body. I forced myself to go out and walk every day. I could barely walk across the room to go to the bathroom, mind you. But I knew the only answer was to "build up" my stamina. Each day, I'd head outside to "exercise." The first day I walked about a half minute at a snail's pace. Wow, what an athlete! But I was so weak I couldn't do more than that. The next day the same, and the next. Then I forced myself to walk a half minute more. A few days later, I added a half minute more. After that strenuous exertion (I'm being sarcastic here!), I'd go in and throw myself onto the couch, exhausted. This slow progress continued, all by sheer determination and will.

In time, however, I became more and more encouraged. I was gaining strength and growing healthier. After many months, I could walk at a good clip for two hours or more without stopping. I've kept at my walking ever since, and now I run a little every day along with my walk.

ber six, the secret to pain-free, low-cost, lifetime fitness: *Learn to love your body in motion!*

Although we're not athletes, we have always enjoyed various forms of movement. Each of us has our favorites: Charity loves swimming and snow skiing, rollerblading and dancing. Being a beach girl, she has even tried surfing! Cynthia was a runner from a young age until the age of thirty-three, when she hurt her knees in an accident. Before that, she would run ten to fifteen miles a day when training for competitions. Now she enjoys long walks, aerobics including step, dancing, and yoga. Sometimes she loves to exercise alone (to think and pray); other days she enjoys the camaraderie of a class with fun, lively music.

Here are several other secrets you can use for success before we launch into active exercise possibilities for you:

Charity Chats

In an interview that I had with John Burch, martial arts instructor and personal trainer at L.A. Urban Fitness in Santa Monica, California, he said visualization was the most important component in a successful image transformation. John should know. He lost fifty-two pounds in twelve weeks! John says you must develop a strong belief system that you're *not* a hopeless case, that you *can* get fit, that it *is* worth the struggle, and that it *will* pay off. He recommends finding a role model and studying his or her life, reading motivating books and magazines, listening to speakers, journaling your thoughts and hopes, and tracking your progress.

One of the most important secrets is *visualization.* Use your "New You" notebook for this purpose. Write down your dreams, goals, and desires for your body and your whole person. Next to your journaling, glue a photo of you in high school or whenever you were in the best shape. If you did it once, you can do it again! You must hold in your head a picture of the person you want to become. That "girl" with glowing health and slim, firm figure. In your notebook, keep a list of all the benefits of regular exercise. Glance over it frequently to remind yourself how much good a little bit of movement will do you.

Healthy Balance secret #6: Learn to love your body in motion.

Here are some of the good things that happen to you when you add the discipline of exercise to your life:

Your *figure* improves as the muscles are toned, and you have more strength and endurance.

You *lose weight* from burning calories and fat, and you charge up your metabolism.

Cynthia Shares

What really works for me is to absolutely love the activity that I choose. For me, it's walking. What draws me to each session is my walking companion. I spend time with Jesus Christ as I stroll. I call my exercise of choice "prayer walking." As I walk, I make the most of my time by strengthening my relationship with God while exercising my heart, lungs, and muscles. Women love the productive idea of doing two things at once, or multitasking as it's called. Besides developing an intimacy with God, prayer walking offers a satisfying way to acquire or maintain an attractive figure. In addition, it's the original Power Walk. I've witnessed amazing answers to prayer as I've "walked and talked" with the Lord.

Your *posture* straightens, not only due to stronger muscles, but also because your *sense of well-being* and *self-esteem* are enhanced.

Your *complexion* glows with good health.

Your *bones* retain their density, and your *joints* become more flexible.

Blood vessels transport life-giving oxygen more efficiently to your whole body, and your *blood pressure* lowers.

Your *heart* is strengthened, and your *heart rate* is reduced.

Your *lungs* expand and process more oxygen.

Your *digestion* and waste removal improve, and your *appetite* is more controlled.

Your *nervous system* relaxes as *stress* is lessened and *depression* lifts.

Sleep comes sooner and is sounder.

Your *brain* sharpens, becoming more alert and able to concentrate.

Charity Chats

I didn't mind the discipline of being on the swim team, because I loved what I was doing. I enjoyed swimming competitively and found that I was good at it. Swimming was the right fit for me athletically. Soon, because swimming was such a perfect lifestyle fit for me, other things began to fit better too . . . like clothes, for instance. Finding the right exercise taught me the joy and rewards of staying active. It's been many years since I swam competitively, but I still love to swim. You can catch me out in the pool getting my exercise several days a week in good weather. I don't have the same rigorous training schedule I once had, but I don't need it. Neither do you. The key is to stay active and move consistently. But you must love the way you choose to move.

And if you include *God* in the activity (as in prayer walking or another activity during which you can also pray, meditate, and memorize Scripture), exercise becomes a complete body and soul prescription for good health and beauty.

It's been said that if exercise were a pill, it would be the most widely prescribed medicine in the world. It's the number one beauty treatment too—and the great thing about exercise is it's free!

If you agree that exercise is important, but you just can't find the time, motivation, or energy, we have some suggestions for you. Supermodel Kim Alexis told us that she dresses in her workout clothes as soon as she hops out of bed. That way, she informs her body, "You're going to exercise today." Try her idea and see if it motivates you. Kim's tricks won't work for me (Cynthia). If I dress in my sweats first thing in the morning, my body thinks, "Lounge around all day." That outfit is just too comfortable! It's better for me to dress in my tightest, most uncomfortable jeans if I want to send my brain and body the message: "Exercise today is mandatory. It's obvious you need it!"

Supercharge for Super Energy

Sometimes we get in a slump in life. For various reasons, we lose our energy and drive. Our metabolism slows down. We gain weight. When we're heavier, we don't feel like moving much. It's a merry-go-round . . . until we devise a plan to jump off.

Here's one way to rev up a stagnant metabolism and gain some energy: In the morning before you start your day, run in place, jump rope, or jump on a minitrampoline for five minutes. It's only five minutes—you can do that, can't you? During your midmorning break and then again at lunch, take a brisk five-minute walk or climb up and down stairs. When you get home from work, hop on the minitramp again for five minutes. We don't recommend exercise before bed—you'll be so charged up you won't fall asleep! But by dividing your workout into small increments throughout your day, you get the benefits of twenty minutes of aerobics without using a large block of time. Research has shown that several short bursts of exercise each day jump-start a sluggish metabolism. As your strength and energy increase, you can lengthen each exercise segment to ten minutes. Think what will happen to your health and figure then!

Want to know how to rev up a sluggish spiritual life? Start exercising your faith! Throughout the day, watch for opportunities to share Christ with friends and colleagues. Notice others' needs. Jesus really is the answer, isn't he?

Study apologetics and the Word of God. Don't hesitate to jump into discussions, even when you're the only Christian defending your faith. Gently, reverently, always be ready to "make a defense to everyone who asks you to give an account for the hope that is in you" (1 Peter 3:15). Spread some of God's love around. Nothing revives a sleepy Christian faster than moving throughout the day as the mouth, hands, and feet of Christ.

Mastering Motivation

As we said in chapter 1, this journey toward the *Healthy and Beautiful Balance* begins with a single step called Desire. Keep the balance yearning burning. Your heart and mind must continually be fed encouraging messages on health, fitness, image, life goals, and true spirituality. Many magazines and books today offer cutting edge information on these subjects. Subscribe to several periodicals or begin a wellness library. You can also find many resources at the public library, including exercise videos to rent. Join an exercise or walking group or a health club if exercising alone bores you. All of us can benefit from the support.

This is so like our spiritual lives. To stay on the narrow path to heaven we need support along the way. That's why Hebrews 10:25 tells us not to forsake fellowshiping together. We've noticed this happening all over the country—Christians are not attending church. Sure you're busy. We all are—too busy actually. Sure it's hard to find a place where you fit in. Your needs must be met. You also must be able to use your spiritual gifts for further growth and edification of the body. It's hard to find the perfect church, and as soon as we find it, the church is imperfect because we're now members! Choose a church (or fellowship of believers) that exalts Jesus Christ as Savior and Lord; one that studies God's Word and believes in living by it; a church that prays and seeks God; a body where members reach out to one another; a church where believers truly enjoy worship and are baptized into the fellowship of Christ; a group that also spreads the gospel and the love of God to the world. When you find a fellowship like this, grab hold and never let go.

Stay excited about your spiritual walk. Read Christian books and magazines. Listen to Christian radio. Begin a new Bible study. Discuss spiritual matters with friends. Attend conferences and retreats. Getting (and staying) in shape spiritually is even more important than physical fitness.

> For more than 75 percent of people in the National Weight Control Registry who have successfully lost weight and kept it off—walking is the answer.
>
> *Prevention—Women's Health Today*

Back to Basics Training

The military knows how to get weak individuals ready for the trenches in a matter of weeks. Just ask any soldier who has been through boot camp. Chad Allen, Cynthia's son and Charity's brother, graduated from the United States Naval Academy, class of 2003. He says he's never done so many push-ups and sit-ups as those he did during Plebe Summer (the Naval Academy's equivalent to boot camp). Chad has assured us that the navy doesn't offer the easy training program that we have here!

Girls just wanna have fun. We know that. But there are also some essential basics to include in your personal exercise regimen. The three most important aspects of physical fitness are *aerobics, strength training,* and *stretching.* In chapter 3 we gave you our nutrition pyramid. We can illustrate exercise with a fitness triangle: aerobics as the base, strength-training next, then stretching. Include these three components on a regular basis and you are guaranteed the best body you've ever had! Let's talk about each of these types of exercise and plan a program for you.

A Cardio Crash Course

Aerobics, or the more recent term, *cardio,* is any repetitive activity that works you hard enough and long enough to get your heart rate up to training level. Haven't paid much attention to your beating heart? Here's how to figure a woman's training heart rate:

Subtract your age from 226. For instance, a 40-year-old's math equation would be:

226 – 40 = 186

186 is her estimated maximum heart rate.

Now calculate the lower and upper numbers of your target zone:

186 × .50 = 93

93 is the low end of her target zone.

186 × .85 = 158

158 is the high end of her target zone.

Somewhere in-between 93 and 158 would be the perfect training heart rate, especially for burning fat. See how your body feels, but don't let it go above or below your calculated numbers.

One way to keep track of your training heart rate is to take your pulse every fifteen minutes per aerobic session. You can do it manually by counting the pulse in your wrist and neck carefully for six seconds, then adding a zero to the number to get your rate for a full minute. For instance, if you count 13 in six seconds, adding the zero makes it 130 for a full minute, a good training heart rate for our forty-year-old female exerciser. (Basically, you are multiplying by ten.)

Another way to keep track of your training heart rate is to use our chart below. The chart shows what a ten-second heart rate would be at 60 percent, 70 percent, and 80 percent maximum training levels for women ages 15 to 80. Copy this page and include it in your "New You" notebook for easy reference. To use it, every fifteen minutes of exercise, stop and check your carotid pulse, at the neck under your jawline. Count for ten seconds, starting with zero, then compare your ten-second rate with the appropriate rates for your age listed in the chart. Try to keep your heart rate steady at 70 percent maximum while exercising—that's where you'll burn the most fat. (Except for pregnant, hypertensive, or very obese ladies. They should exercise at 50–60 percent.) As you continue training aerobically, you'll grow accustomed to how your body feels when it's getting just the right amount of exercise.

Target Heart Rates

Age	60 percent	70 percent	80 percent
15	21	24	27
20	20	23	27
25	19	23	26
30	19	22	25

Age	60 percent	70 percent	80 percent
35	19	22	25
40	18	21	24
45	18	20	23
50	17	20	23
55	17	19	22
60	16	19	21
65	16	18	21
70	15	18	20
75	15	17	19
80	14	16	19

Aerobics (a name given this type of exercise in the sixties by the king of cardio, Dr. Kenneth Cooper) means "with air." You want the activity to force you to breathe in more oxygen than usual. By no means are you to be gasping for air, however! Just a steady in-and-out flow deep into the lungs is what you're after. It should feel refreshing—at least when you're done!

Fun Unlimited

This is the era of choice. We hear it all the time: a woman's right to choose. Be pro-choice. Let's use this motto for God's kingdom! Yes, you have the right to choose—to choose to do good, to love, to live healthy. Of the many delicious whole foods in the world, lucky you, you get to choose new ones each day. And of all the fun activities available in the world to use for fitness, you get to now choose a favorite. To aid in your decision making, ask yourself a few easy questions:

Do you prefer indoor or outdoor activities?
Do you have any health problems that prohibit sun exposure? Or any health problems, period?

Is your main objective to firm muscles, improve health, lose fat, or do all three?

Do you like to exercise alone, with a partner, or in groups?

Does music motivate you? Do trainers and group leaders challenge or intimidate you?

Do you have lots of time for exercise? Or do you need to do your "daily dozen" in a matter of minutes?

Usually aerobics will mean weight-bearing exercises, but bicycling and swimming also count if sustained for at least twenty minutes. There are other activities that get your heart rate up quickly, but they don't last long enough to be aerobic!

Some pleasant outdoor choices that can be done alone, with a partner, or in groups include walking, hiking, running, in-line skating, swimming, bicycling, rowing, cross-country skiing, and snowshoeing. These activities get your heart rate up, burn some fat, work your heart, lungs, and circulation, and use approximately 300 calories per half hour of exercise (except for walking, which uses 150 calories per half hour, and running, at 350 calories per half hour). Which ones sound fun to you?

There are some advantages in choosing one of these workouts. Outdoor activities can give you a new perspective. The simple act of stepping out into the sunshine and fresh air lifts spirits and chases cares away. Don't exercise in the heat of the day, though, and always wear sunscreen and preferably a hat when exercising in sunlight. In addition, sunglasses prevent those little crinkly squint lines. They also hinder passersby from recognizing you when you're out limping along on your fifth mile!

Indoor cardio choices include aerobic dance, step aerobics, spinning (a new type of stationary cycling), circuit weight training, jumping rope, karate/tae kwon do, racquetball, stationary bike, rowing machine, stairclimber, ski machine, and treadmill. These exercises can also be done alone, with a partner, or in groups. Some involve little expense. If you choose to do aerobic dance in the privacy of your home, all you need is an exercise video or some music. Others require various levels of commitment and cost. Health club memberships can be pricey, but they may be worth the expense to keep you consistent. These workouts challenge your heart, lungs, and muscles, also burning fat and calories (between 200–350 per half hour of exercise). Indoor exercises have the advantage of being private and weatherproof. And if you have a tendency to boredom, you can watch the news or read a magazine while on a machine. A schedule that works well plus keeps you committed is to choose several sports or machines and alternate them.

Whenever we speak to groups on this subject, the same questions come up frequently. Here are the answers to some of the most common queries.

Are warm-ups and cooldowns really that important?

Yes! You wouldn't think of starting the car on a cold day without warming it up, would you? (Well, at least not if your husband was watching!) The same is true with your body. Warm-ups need not be difficult. Just begin with five minutes of easy walking, then pick up the pace or begin your activity. In fact, on days when I (Cynthia) am not feeling energetic, this is how I talk myself into exercising. I tell myself, *Just do five minutes.* In five minutes, I'm full of energy and in a good mood, ready to go the second mile! Those who warm up are less prone to injuries. The warm-up sends blood to the muscles in use, preparing them for the workout ahead.

Cooldowns can be just as easy. When you've worked your heart at target rate for at least twenty minutes, cool down with an easy walk. Continued movement for five minutes prevents the blood from pooling in your legs and feet. It also cools down your body temperature and slows your heart rate and breathing to normal. Trust us, you'll look forward to that cooldown walk.

How often must I work out?

The question should be rephrased to "How often do I *get* to work out?" Or "How often will I *want* to work out once I'm addicted to it?" As often as your schedule allows! As far as training results, you need to exercise five or six days a week. The minimum would be three days a week, but that won't contribute to much weight loss.

How long do I need to work out each session to lose weight?

Aim for forty-five minutes of exercise six days a week, with one day off for rest and muscle renewal. Most of each session should be spent at your target heart rate. You can do the math to figure how much weight you'll lose. If you burn 500 extra calories a day exercising, it will take seven days to lose a pound of fat. If you want faster weight loss, exercise more (both in the morning and evening), or deduct 500 calories from each day's menus. That will give you the recommended two pounds a week loss of fat. Anything more is water weight.

What should I do for more of a challenge?

If you've been exercising for a while, you may want to increase your fitness level. You can add interval training to your exercise session by interspersing short, intense bursts of activity with the slower, sustained movement. Start with short intervals of intense exercise—fifteen to thirty seconds—and build up from there.

I (Cynthia) do interval training with our dog, Spike. I walk, then jog. Then I up the ante. When I holler, "Go, Spike, go!" our cocker knows he can take off. He gallops (or whatever it is that dogs do), ears flying, as fast as he can go under constraint of his leash. And that's the catch: I'm holding the leash, so I have to sprint too. I lengthen my stride and really run. Heavy breathing and all that. When I've had enough, I yell, "Slow down, Spike!" We walk for a while, then jog, then do the routine over until my exercise time is up. It's a great workout and lots of fun . . . until Spike decides to dart in front of me and I bite the dust. Every sport has its hazards!

Ready for a challenge? Take on some hills! Walking, running, biking, and hiking all accommodate themselves to hill climbing. Race up, jog down, race up, jog down. "Who needs more challenge than that?" you'll be wondering after a few minutes of this routine.

Speaking of racing, add some fun competition to your exercise routine. Invite another runner (biker, swimmer, climber) to join you. (They will take the place of Spike in your workout, but don't tell them they're replacing a dog!) After warm-ups, begin your exercise, then race to a designated stop. But don't stop there. Continue your reduced pace, then race again. The winner is rewarded with a few extra calories burned! Enjoy stimulating conversation while you cool down. Then head to the minimart for a bottle of cooled spring water or fruit juice.

If you love aerobic dance, it's easy to pick up the pace. Find livelier music, something that gets your toes tapping, your feet stomping, your hands clapping. No one has to tell you to move when music with a beat is playing. It comes naturally!

What happens if I take a few weeks off?

Fat happens! Just kidding, but researchers have found that cardiovascular improvements diminish within weeks of discontinuing exercise. Even on vacation, try to walk, exercise in the hotel gym, or do some yoga or stretching in your room. This is a commitment for life!

But the commitment need not be a burden. Hours in the gym are unnecessary (except for professional bodybuilders). Anything more than an hour proves that the quest for fitness has become a hobby or maybe an obsession. Your goal is to choose some enjoyable activities and then do one of them for a half hour a day (twenty minutes minimum). For you, it might be putting on a CD of Middle Eastern music, grabbing a veil, and twirling around the room as an imaginary belly dancer. Believe it or not, I (Cynthia) have taken a belly-dance class. I learned a lot about the dance in addition to its steps and moves. Originally belly dancing was symbolic movement that women performed only in the company of other women. You don't need an audience of either sex to try it, however. Lock the door, pull the drapes, and shimmy those hips. You'll burn lots of calories and firm muscles with this ancient art form.

Find an activity you love. It needs to be simple, easily accessible, and affordable, and it must be appealing. The "no pain, no gain" theory went out with the eighties. Don't you return over and over to the things you enjoy? Do something fun, just keep moving! When you find an activity you love, old or new, you'll never want to take time off from it.

Strength Training

We know you have no desire to become a female Arnold Schwarzenegger. But the weight room has always been the place to discover the Body Beautiful, be it yours or someone else's. Aerobics will help burn calories and fat. It firms muscles moderately. But nothing can beat weight lifting for building and shaping the muscles of your body. Let's not just *talk* about buns of steel—the weight room is the place to actually pick up a pair!

In addition, there are also several good health reasons to begin a strength-training program. Research over the past few years indicates that working out with weights improves the body on the inside too. Look at these benefits:

Stay strong. If you don't exercise, you'll lose 30–40 percent of your muscle capacity by age sixty-five. That's almost half your strength! Two-thirds of the great-grandmas in America can't lift anything heavier than ten pounds. Grandmas, your latest grandbaby already weighs thirteen! Please don't think this is another unavoidable effect of aging. Use it or lose it, sister! Muscles that go unused become weaker and weaker. They were made to be worked long into those golden years.

Weight lifting with dumbbells (and we're not talking about the crowd you exercise with!) is a more pleasant form of training than piano lifting or boat towing with your teeth. Machines also provide appropriate resistance. Sessions with either should be included for muscle building and maintenance.

Build strong bones. For years, weight-bearing exercise (aerobics) was thought to be the way to maintain your bone mass. Now studies show that resistance training will do the same thing. At age thirty-five or so, most of us begin to lose up to 1 percent of our bone per year. After menopause, the loss is even greater. When you lift weights, you stress the bone, stimulating its growth. Combine weight training with aerobics and the *Healthy Balance* diet, and you have a plan to battle osteoporosis.

More balance, fewer injuries. As you strengthen muscles in every section of your body, your balance improves. You are less apt to fall. In addition, as the muscles increase, new circulatory paths are created, bringing a fresh blood supply to heal injured areas. Tightened muscles hold your head high, shoulders back, and tummy flat. Improved posture gives you a new sense of confidence. You look and feel like a balanced person!

Metabolic magic. This is the best discovery of all! Weight training revs up your metabolism to burn more calories, even when you're resting! Your resting metabolism is the number of calories needed to maintain your body's important functions like pumping blood and digesting food. Muscles need more energy. The bigger and stronger your muscles, the more calories you will burn. Now that's not an excuse to eat more, but it will make your body more efficient. On the

---

Charity Chats

Richard Culp, my grandfather, is a perfect example of the benefits of keeping in shape. In his mid-seventies, he has the strength of a much younger man because he refuses to become idle. He has continued his second career as a hunting club manager in rural northern California. This outdoor work requires much heavy lifting, which he insists on doing himself (he is as strong as a bull, and just as bullheaded). He is no Jack LaLanne. When the motor on the duck hunters' boat goes out, he doesn't tow it in with his teeth. (Jack actually did this on his eightieth birthday! Whoopee—what a way to celebrate!) But he is assured of his own strength. Not long ago when asked to help move a piano, he insisted on doing it himself. We prayed for protection (both for him and the piano!), and the job got done with no resulting hernias.

other side of the mirror, if you don't build up muscle mass, you'll burn fewer calories no matter how little you eat. Not a pretty picture, is it?

Temple Maintenance

Don't worry. You won't end up as a competitor in the World Wrestling Federation. Women don't have the hormonal or structural makeup to become as big as men. If you work out with weights consistently, say three times a week, every other day, you will see a huge difference in about six weeks. But not in size. The improvements will show up as tight, contracted muscles (even those Chicken Arms we've complained about!), better shape, better balance and posture, smaller clothing size, and possibly a slight weight gain.

Weight gain? Count me out, you say. But muscle weighs more than fat. And it looks firmer, tighter, and smaller. Plus, as you stay on the *Healthy Balance* plan, decreasing your calories and upping your exercise, you'll be losing fat and increasing muscle. Don't worry about the scale. If you've been overweight from extra fat, you should see a drop in pounds. But notice how your clothes fit. Look in the mirror. Do you see a difference in your shape? Disregard set weights on charts. How do you feel? Live your life to please God, not others. If you like the way you look, even if you are large, thank God. Eat healthy and exercise for cardiovascular fitness. Forget today's impossible standards! Just think if we were living back during the Renaissance—plump women were in vogue. Trends come and go.

Our bodies are the temples of the Holy Spirit, according to 1 Corinthians 6:19. Love yourself as God loves you. Eat and exercise to maintain his temple—your body—and you'll find a body balance that's easy to live with.

Proverbia strengthened areas of her busy body. For obvious reasons, she didn't have much time, but it really doesn't take much time to keep your muscles firm and strong. Unless you're planning to enter that bodybuilder's contest, fifteen minutes to a half hour three times a week is all you need to be toned. Actress Raquel Welch, who is well into her sixties and still turning heads, claims that she works out for two hours a day, six days a week. We don't want to spend that much time on it, do you? We have better things to do with our time. There's a visible difference between Raquel's value system and ours. The apostle Paul revealed that he whipped his body into shape, mastering it. However, "bodily discipline is only of little profit, but godliness is profitable for all things, since it holds promise for the present and also for the life to come," he explained in 1 Timothy 4:8. So that's why Raquel has the two-hour-a-day figure and we have the ten-minute-a-day bodies. Our values are different. At least, that's our excuse! But no more excuses—the following section provides an easy fifteen-minute conditioning routine to firm and strengthen problem spots.

Weight Training without Weights

There are many books on the market that instruct you how to strength train using dumbbells, barbells, and whole-body machines. There are clubs and gyms that also offer instruction. As we finish this section, we'd like to offer you simple resistant exercises that will work you out without added weights. Plus this workout is absolutely free! George Foreman, champion heavyweight boxer and now king of the portable grill empire, doesn't use weights when he trains. Instead, he uses the resistance of his own body, and that's what you'll do here. By using the lighter load and doing more repetitions (reps), you tone your muscles instead of building bulk. Plus you'll have all the strength necessary for your everyday life. You'll need a mat of some sort (or a folded quilt) and a chair. Begin with the suggested number of reps (or even fewer if you've never exercised. It only takes one attempt to build new muscle tissue!) and rest for thirty seconds between sets. Consecutive repetitions of one exercise defines a set.

> Through the centuries, plump was pleasing. Extra body weight proved that you had the money to eat more than enough. At the turn of the twentieth century, thin became "in." The wealthy ate in an elegant, controlled, leisurely fashion. Perhaps we should hope for a cultural curves revival. Larger women may be riding the crest of the next wave of popular style!

We'll use a chair as a prop for the first part of our workout.

> *For Hips, Thighs, and Buns:* Leg Lifts. Stand behind a chair and hold on to its back. While pressing your pelvis into the back of the chair, lift your right leg behind you with pointed toe. Continue to lift your right leg with pointed toe for 9 more repetitions; then contract your toes and lift 10 times (or work up to this amount if just starting out). Turn and hang on to the chair's back with your left hand. Standing straight (don't lean to the left or right), raise and lower right leg out to the side, 10 reps with pointed toe, then 10 lifts with contracted toes. Only raise your leg about two feet or so. Repeat these exercises for your left leg. Work up to about 15 or 20 reps. (This exercise can also be done at the kitchen sink.) If you want, you can add weights to your legs as you build strength. Weight training of any sort will build lean body mass, which in turn revs up your metabolism. This routine won't give you buns of steel, but it will tighten that little tush of yours!
>
> *For Buttocks:* Bun Lifts. Sit on chair, holding on to edge. Stretch out legs and raise and lower buns. Tighten gluteus muscles with each lift and hold. Do 8 reps.
>
> *For Triceps (Chicken Arms):* Chair Lift. Stay on the edge of a sturdy chair. Place hands near your buttocks, fingers facing out. Stretch your legs out in front of you and lower your body until your buns nearly touch the floor. Hold this position for two seconds, then lift back up, using the muscles in the back of your arms. Feel them working? Repeat this lifting and lowering motion 3–5 times. Do 3 sets. This is a difficult move

for most women. Build reps up gradually and rest between sets.

For Abs: Chair Crunch. Sit in the chair. Scoot your bottom to the edge of the seat and hang on to the edge with your hands. With bent knees, lift legs up to chest, then lower, straightening legs but not letting them touch the floor. Back up to chest, then straight out again. Start with 5 reps. Work up to 20, contracting stomach muscles continually.

Reclining Windmill. Lay on the mat and continue your ab work. Lie flat on your back, legs outstretched, arms cradling back of head. Simultaneously, bring knees up and lift head and torso until elbows touch knees. Repeat 5–10 times. Rest, then do another set. You can vary this exercise by touching opposite elbow and knee in a bicycle motion.

For Arms, Shoulders, and Chest: The Reliable Push-up. Roll over and get on all fours. Place hands shoulder-width apart, fingers pointing out. Lower upper body almost to the mat. Hold, then raise up to the starting position. Repeat 4 times. Do 2 sets. Build up reps and sets as your strength increases.

To Cool Down: Reward Time. Collapse on mat and finish with a long, slow stretch.

These exercises are firming up muscle groups. If you have weight to lose, calorie and fat reduction is a must. It's been said that if spot reducing worked, people who chew gum would have skinny faces! We're aiming for total body (and soul) fitness here. Make exercise as much a part of your daily habits as brushing your teeth. In a matter of weeks you'll be in great shape if you also add some gentle aerobics to your routine.

One of the best fitness plans we've found is to turn the above routine into a circuit program with strength training and aerobics. I (Cynthia) turn on the news and begin my workout by jumping on a minitramp. When I get tired of that after several minutes, I hit the mat for some ab work and push-ups. When those exhaust me, I hop back onto the trampoline. In a few more minutes, I stop jumping and do the chair routines. Back and forth, back and forth, between the mat, the chair, and the minitramp, not resting in between (you should never rest more than thirty seconds in circuit training). Sometimes instead of watching TV, I put on lively music or listen to a Bible tape. A half hour of this keeps my heart rate high, burns calories, firms muscles, and I'm never bored. When I'm finished, I enjoy a brief, relaxed stretch.

Stretching

The last aspect of your fitness triangle is stretching. A soothing stretch is a great way to cool down at the end of your aerobics or weight-training session. Regular stretching improves posture, corrects muscle imbalances, soothes painful areas of the body, gives you a supple figure with elongated muscles, and improves your flexibility. Your flexibility is determined by how mobile your joints are. How easily can you move, stretch, and bend? We all start life with incredible abilities. Have you seen babies manage to place their tasty toes into their tiny mouths? Newborns are very flexible. We all spend nine months curled up into a little ball. It takes us a lifetime to grow stiff and tight, unbendable and inflexible.

The American College of Sports Medicine recommends flexibility training three times a week. These sessions need not be long; five to ten minutes will stretch the whole body. Hold each stretch for ten to thirty seconds and repeat each three to five times for best results.

Here are some rules to remember as you stretch:

Move slowly. Hurrying is the antithesis to stretching.

Feel the stretch—but not the pain.

Hold each stretch for ten counts. Or at least work up to that.

Don't bounce or jerk. This contracts the muscle instead of elongating it. Plus you risk injuring yourself. Torn muscles take weeks and months to heal.

Breathe deeply. Stretching can actually increase your lung capacity if you concentrate on breathing deeply into your diaphragm. The increase in oxygen is beneficial. And deep breathing calms you down, releasing stress and tension from your body.

Work flexibility exercises into your daily life. Does a cat have a special time for stretching? No, she does it whenever she feels like her body needs it. A good, slow stretch will wake you up in the morning. Remember that stretching energizes you. When you're behind your desk in the afternoon or while driving on a trip, stop and take a stretch break.

Flex Your Options

You might want to look into several effective methods of stretching. Hatha yoga (the physical aspect of yoga) has been around for five thousand years. Originating in India, this quiet form of exercise is very different from bouncy, noisy American aerobics classes. In yoga, you proceed through a series of poses, or asanas, all the while breathing deeply, focusing your mind, entering into the stretch. The asanas work and stretch every muscle group. In addition, your spine is kept pliable.

To begin yoga practice, select a book from a bookstore or the library. It helps if you have pictures to look at. The instructions will tell you things to be cautious of in addition to steps for each asana. You can also purchase video classes taught by nationally famous yoga instructors. If you really want to get into it, real classes are available from private teachers or through groups like the YMCA and health clubs. Visit the class first to be sure it's for beginners. Watch the instructor. Does he or she give personal instruction and correction to each student? This is what you're looking for, so choose a class that meets your needs. Does the yoga teacher present the postures without Eastern religion propaganda? This can get tiresome for a Christian who only joined for a good stretch. Choose a class that meets your personal body-and-soul needs.

Pilates (pronounced pih-law-teez) is the latest buzzword in fitness. Surely you've heard of it (unless you've been living in a cave!). The stars are always bragging about their Pilates workouts or instructors. Perhaps you've wondered what Pilates is. I (Cynthia) was very inquisitive as I heard reports of miracle bodies being molded by this current exercise trend. I checked out a Pilates class at a local health club but didn't want to pay the price (Pilates classes can be very expensive!). So I bought several books to educate myself. What I've read is that Pilates works the important muscle groups in the center of the body, your core as it's called in

Pilates. (Remember Proverbia's loin workouts!) Your abs, lower back, thighs, and buttocks are challenged intensely. The method was created by Joseph Pilates, a gymnast, who used it to rehabilitate dancers. Like yoga, Pilates works the mind as well as the body (through intense focus and concentration). The moves require much deliberate effort, and you are continually working to new levels. Pilates machines are also available to further stretch and strengthen your whole body.

Here we offer a simple stretch routine that you can do after aerobics or weight training:

Stand tall on the mat and roll your head in a complete circle, stretching neck muscles.

Reach right arm to the sky and hold. Reach left arm and hold. Then both arms.

Clasp hands behind back. Bring arms up behind back, then above head as you bend over from the waist. Hold steady (no bouncing) for 10–15 seconds. Increase as your flexibility improves.

Hands on hips, bend slightly backward, pushing hips forward. Hold.

Slowly bend at the waist and touch toes. Hold.

Straddle mat. With right arm overhead, bend sideways to the left, stretching right side of body. Hold. Stretch other side. Stand up straight again.

Raise both hands over head and slowly bend at waist to touch toes again. Hold.

Slowly lower your body into a squat. Then roll back onto mat, clasping knees.

Cynthia Shares

I first tried Hatha yoga after the birth of my first child, Charity. I had been a runner before her birth (even running my miles the day of her delivery). But I found myself housebound once the baby came. I bought a book on yoga and with limited knowledge began a daily series of asanas. It was all very experimental. I had always believed if exercise wasn't strenuous, it wasn't working. But within six weeks, my lung capacity was as good as when I ran regularly, and my body was firm and supple. I had that long, lean look (after the baby fat disappeared, that is!). I was sold! I've been doing some yoga (minus the chants and incense) ever since. I use this quiet, focused time for real communication with my Creator instead. The prayer is good for my soul while the slow stretches are good for my body. The healthy balance!

Lie on back, knees bent. Lift hips up to ceiling and hold. Lower to mat.

Lie on mat. Raise up and bend toward feet. Grasp toes. Hold. Bend right knee and place right foot near groin. Stretch toward left foot, touching toe with hand, and hold. Bend left knee and place left foot near groin. Stretch toward right foot, touching toe with hand, and hold.

Sit with legs in wide V. Bend toward left foot, hold. Bend toward right foot, hold. Bend toward middle of V, hold.

Legs back together, bend at waist and touch toes. Hold.

Roll back onto mat. While lying on back, lift legs, then hips over head. Support with your hands (bend elbows). Lower toes to floor behind head, if possible (if not, do as much of the stretch as you can; you'll get there). Hold. Lower legs slowly back to mat (supporting body with hands). Use stomach muscles to control speed of legs.

Lie completely still on mat, arms and legs outstretched, and breath deeply 10 times. Enjoy the peaceful feeling of a good stretch!

Cynthia's son Caleb is a wonderful athlete. His sports are football, basketball, and track. His coaches emphasize a stretching routine similar to this one before each event. Caleb is now a faithful stretcher—after sitting out several weeks with a torn hamstring. Don't forget to stretch!

Be sure to stretch yourself spiritually too. Move out of your comfort zone into new avenues of service for the Lord. Notice the peaceful, fulfilled feeling you get!

A perfect *Healthy Balance* plan would be to do at least a half hour of circuit weight training on Mondays, Wednesdays, and Fridays. Then do aerobics like walking, jogging, or biking on Tuesdays, Thursdays, and one weekend day. The rest day builds and restores your muscles. Alternating activities keeps you from becoming bored, plus the cross training works all your muscle groups, increasing strength and endurance. Add a little stretching at the end of your aerobic sessions, and you're good for the gold!

8

Geared Up for Fitness

We really don't need anything but determination to pursue health and physical conditioning. And the only possession you need for spiritual fitness is your Bible. However, things often go more easily if we have some tried-and-true tools to assist us in our diligent efforts. One of the best tools you can use to get fit and stay fit is your "New You" notebook. I have found this to be true in my (Cynthia's) own life. When I am listing the foods I eat each day, tallying the calorie count, visually eyeing my poor choices or celebrating my good ones, I stay committed to my nutritional plan. When I jot down my daily exercise, I feel successful. When I record and date the lessons that God is teaching me, I never forget them. They are always there for me when I need to be reminded of his faithfulness, whether it's one month later or ten years later.

Your "New You" notebook, featuring you as its star, will keep you on track and assist you in the visualization of your goals. We can't state it enough: Desire, commitment, and perseverance are the keys to success! Visualization and fantasizing often have negative connotations, but Dr. Charles Stanley of Atlanta asserts that God created our minds with their ability to visualize. "Use fantasizing for good," he says.

"Imagine yourself to greatness!" In a sermon on the subject of visualization, Dr. Stanley explained this more fully:

> The mind that can destroy you and cast you down is the same mind that can catapult you to great success. Stamp indelibly upon your mind the image of the person you want to become. Get that image fixed in your mind. Don't let it fade away. Ignore negative comments—you are going somewhere! Remind yourself, *God is changing the way I think (positive, successful, reaching my goals, expecting miracles). He is changing the way I look and feel (healthy, fit, peaceful, relaxed). He is changing my spirit to be like his.* The "how" is not your issue, but God's. Have faith![1]

Dr. Stanley recommends titling a sheet of paper "The Person I Want to Become." Write down every detail of that beautiful, shapely, charming, healthy, educated, godly person that you want to grow into. Jot down single words or phrases. Don't belabor the exercise. Keep that page in a section of your "New You" notebook. Study this list daily. We move toward the things we think about. Tell yourself, *Anything I think about long enough becomes my reality. I need to be careful of what I'm thinking, or I may move in a direction I don't want to go.* Charles Stanley insists that if you don't think about it, you won't become anything but what you already are. If you write it down, he says, your life will change. Focus your attention on what you desire to become instead of who you are now, instead of on your failures, weaknesses, and fears about the future.

Think positively about yourself:

I'll look differently.
I'll act differently.

I'll talk differently.
I'll dress and drive differently.
I'll live differently.

A whole new you awaits the expectant world. Don't make the world wait too long!

Your "New You" Notebook

Studies reveal that dieters who journal (recording daily menus, calorie counts, emotional eating triggers, and exercise strategies) lose the most weight. We covered the "New You" notebook extensively in "Makeover Miracles," chapter 2 of *The Beautiful Balance for Body and Soul,* but we'll explain again here briefly how you can make your own life-changing notebook. Buy an inexpensive loose-leaf binder, the kind that you carried around in high school.

> I dwell in possibility.
>
> Emily Dickinson

Choose your favorite color. (Cynthia uses a regular-sized green [to symbolize growth] notebook that holds lined paper 8½ x 11 inches. Charity prefers a smaller 5 x 7 version that travels more easily.) We both like the binders with the clear vinyl on the front cover so we can display our motivational pictures and favorite famous quotes.

Inside the notebook's covers, use dividers to categorize your notebook however you desire. Here are some section suggestions: Dreams and goals, Beauty (hair, skin, face, fashion), Figure (exercise program, food journal, health pursuits), Soul Care, Miscellaneous (list of books to read, movies to watch, events to attend; a calendar, addresses and phone numbers of friends). Your "New You" notebook should be as individual as you are. Be creative! Use colored pens and markers. Cut and paste pictures and motivational sayings from magazines and newspapers. Save poems that inspire you. The notebook is yours—an expression of who you are and who you are becoming. You are the celebrity here, so be sure to shine!

Tool Time

Actually, you don't need anything but your own body to begin exercising. But there are several tools that will enhance your training sessions and several more that you can purchase as motivational treats. If you wonder where to find the extra dollars, set aside the money you'd normally spend on junk food. Save up until you can buy some trendy, comfortable exercise togs or a piece of helpful equipment. In addition, after you've been exercising for a period of time, you may want to occasionally buy books, videos, clothing, and equipment to keep your interest, excitement, and commitment high.

> The Lord told the prophet Habakkuk, "Record the vision and inscribe it on tablets, that the one who reads it may run."
>
> Habakkuk 2:2

Footloose and Fancy-Free

Shoes are the most important piece of exercise equipment. Good shoes support your body weight, cushioning the impact on your feet, ankles, knees, and hips when running or exercising. Select shoes with plenty of cushion. Big gals will want more height in the heel, which indicates more midsole foam. Jog around the store in your exercise shoes, preferably on tile, before you take them home. The toebox (section for your toes) shouldn't pinch, and there should be a half inch between the end of the shoe and your big toe. If the shoe is too loose at the heel, you can get blisters. Women with narrow feet can wear an extra pair of socks if they can't find a shoe with perfect fit. Also, don't wear your laces too long. You can cut them to the right length and tie knots at the ends or use lace locks. Experience has taught us that a too-long shoelace can trip a runner when she least expects it!

If you can only afford one thing, buy decent running or sport-specific shoes. The rule is buy running shoes for running, jogging and walking, stair climbing, and circuit weight training; buy sport-specific shoes for the sport (like tennis shoes for tennis), or buy cross trainers for aerobics, step aerobics, and aerobic dancing.

Clothes with Class

Would you ever exercise in your corset and skintight leather pants? Of course not! Why? Comfort rules! And of course, you wouldn't be able to move like you want to (although Madonna seems to be the rare exception!). It's important to wear comfortable, stretchy, weather-appropriate clothing when exercising.

How do you feel when you walk into the health club wearing a stained, tight, torn leotard or dated gym clothes? Like Cinderella at the ball after midnight? All eyes on you for all the wrong reasons! Fashionable, colorful exercise outfits will add fun to your workouts, supporting your commitment and enthusiasm for the next session.

Down under, you also need support. Be sure that your bra has the proper lift for the size of your breasts. Sport bras are especially made for exercising. Compression-style bras hold the breasts inward toward the chest wall (similar to how they wrapped women in the olden days). These only work for small- or medium-sized women. Full-breasted women will prefer the encapsulation-style bras that hold breasts steady with seams or wire. Straps should be strong, with appropriate elasticity. You don't want your undergarments to chafe around the middle either. Wear your correct size.

Your exercise outfits will greatly enhance your fitness sessions. Purchase tops and bottoms in fabrics that move well, breathe, and dry quickly when wet, like polyester, spandex, cotton blends, wool, and wool blends. When trying clothes on, give yourself plenty of room to move and breathe. And of course, choose your favorite, energy-producing colors!

Don't forget the importance of socks. When color coordinated, they complete your outfit. They also cushion your feet and ankles and reduce rubbing at the sides and tops of your feet. Look for wool and wool blends, nylon, and cotton blends.

Weather Wear

If you exercise outdoors, you will want to dress for the weather. In the summer, it's not hard to figure out what to wear. As little as the law (and morality) will allow you, right? Just don't forget your sunscreen, sunglasses, and when possible a hat.

In the cold of winter, your first inclination is to bundle up. But five minutes into your workout, you're sweating bullets with nowhere to drop that woolly mammoth faux fur jacket! Instead, try layering. Sweats or exercise pants on the bottom (and if you live in the snow, perhaps also leggings), long-sleeved sweatshirt or sweater layered over a long-sleeved T-shirt on top. You can strip off the top layer as you get overheated and tie it around your waist. Heat escapes from your head and feet. Wool socks and a knitted cap on your head will alleviate that problem.

In Step with Time

You will want an easy-to-read wristwatch for timing exercise sessions. (Go for time, not miles, at least a half hour per session.) Make sure the numbers are big enough to read. In addition, you may want a watch face that lights up for early morning and evening workouts. Use the second hand to check your heart rate. Every fifteen minutes, stop or walk slowly and count your pulse for six seconds. Add a zero to the number and you have your heart rate for one minute. If it's not up to training level, pick up the pace. If you're exercising too hard, slow it down.

Heart rate monitors are handy little gadgets to keep you exercising at a productive level of intensity. They do the figuring for you. Some monitors are a strap system worn below the breasts at your bra line. You want it to fit snugly but comfortably. Make sure the numbers are visible and readable. A single read (the heart rate only) on the face is larger; the more info, the smaller the numbers. You can also buy wristwatches that track your pulse.

The Best Choice

The treadmill is the most frequently used exercise machine. Walking is an easy activity that nearly everyone can do. On the machine, you can walk in front of the TV or while reading a book. With a treadmill, you have no excuses. You exercise rain or shine, night or day. And the machine keeps you at training intensity—there's no slipping into a slowdown unless you program it into the machine!

When you shop for your treadmill, buy a machine with a minimum horsepower of 1½ or 2. That way, if you get energetic and break out into a run, the machine will accommodate you. A treadmill with elevation change capabilities adds to the variety of your workouts. You'll want railings on the front and sides to hang on to. A flexible deck and smooth belt action keep the machine running smoothly and you running smoothly on it. Decide which computer programs you want on the display panel: calories expended, elevation levels, programmed workouts, heart rate monitor, or whatever your machine can display.

Before you head out of the athletic store, ask several more questions: How much noise does the machine make when running? How much room does it take? Is the walking area on it long enough for your stride? What is its maximum speed and maximum elevation? Does it have any specialty features that you want, like a cup holder or a book or magazine rack?

Try the treadmill of your choice out at the store before you buy. And don't be suckered into one of those nonelectric, human-powered contraptions. It will end up in the garage collecting dust or be someone else's bargain at your next yard sale!

Speaking of garage sales, another good piece of exercise equipment can be found at them or many secondhand shops: the minitrampoline. One unique feature of the minitramp is its gravity affect. This activates the lymph glands and keeps the lymph fluid flowing through the body.

Why Weight?

Dumbbells. Not you, of course. These are my exercise tools of choice (Charity). I use five-pound and ten-pound weights three times a week to firm up my upper body. I do three sets of twelve reps each of shoulder presses, chest presses, pectoral flies, and tricep lifts. Occasionally I use ankle weights when I do leg lifts as well. The added resistance works like a charm to firm up my muscles without too much torture!

For Flexible Fun

Exercise balls. These are great for support while working your abs. Your body beckons more muscles to help stay balanced on the ball. You can do incredible stretches, bending in ways you never thought possible. Many chiropractors recommend exercise balls for bad backs, unbalanced sides of the body, and gentle stretching of tight areas. Exercise balls come in four sizes. Choose the size appropriate for you:

If you are 4'7" to 5' use a 45-centimeter ball.
If you are 5'1" to 5'6" use a 55-centimeter ball.
If you are 5'7" to 5'11" use a 65-centimeter ball.
If you are over 6' use a 75-centimeter ball.

The more expensive balls are stronger and more durable, plus they often come with explanatory books or videos. If a foot or hand pump is not included, be sure to purchase one. Save your breath for exercising, not blowing up balls!

Trainers Who Come to You

Speaking of videos, nothing can be a better investment than several good exercise videos. Be sure the instructor's personality and style meshes with yours. She should lead you through a brief warm-up, an aerobics session of at least twenty minutes, maybe some spot toning, then a relaxing cooldown, all the while keeping you energized with her encouragement and lively background music. Currently our favorite video instructors are Leslie Sansone, Becky Tirabassi, and Joannie Greggains. But usually we will just pick up videos for a dollar or two at secondhand shops. That way if we don't like the workouts, we can donate the videos to the library without feeling buyers' remorse.

A Little Help from an Old Friend

Girdles. If all else fails, buy a girdle! Just kidding, of course. When did girdles go out of style? Enquiring minds want to know! They were handy in a pinch (and we mean, pinch!).

The 1940s and '50s brought us a revolution in women's couture. It was possible to look fashionably fit without ever lacing up a jogging shoe. Similar to the iron corsets of Queen Victoria's day, this invention promised not only tiny waists but flat tummies and firm hips too. The rubber/latex girdle had become a recommended addition to any stylish woman's wardrobe. I (Cynthia) remember my grandmother and mother squeezing into those rubbery contraptions, tugging, shimmying, until they were stuffed into them like sausages. But the effects were amazing—bulges gone, stomachs smoothed, thighs tamed. Silk dresses slipped easily over controlled figures. The viewing public was offered an illusion of fitness.

Under the physical facade, however, the poor woman was pinched and pulled until breathless. And when she took the thing off, well, I think that's where the saying "Let it all hang out!" came from. In the late '60s and early '70s, women threw out not only their girdles, but some did away with their bras too! They didn't want any type of constriction. A fitness fad took over the nation. Some trends are detrimental, but this was a wave that benefited America's population. Now we women know that strengthening our God-given girdle, like Proverbia does, is the healthy, natural way to look slim and fit.

Tools for the Soul

Just as there is equipment for physical training, there are tools to train the soul. As Christians, we must train ourselves to see everything with a spiritual eye. Charles Stanley calls this "the third eye of the believer." We're not talking about a multi-eyed, Bible-packing monster here! Instead, we must develop discerning hearts and minds to live effectively for Christ. Remember, as a man thinks in his heart, so is he (Prov. 23:7). The direction that our hearts and minds are feeling and thinking is the direction that our body and actions will take us.

In Dr. Stanley's message on faith, he refers to Moses, who had this "third eye." Hebrews 11 talks about how the Hebrew leader persevered through the wilderness journey, tolerating the demands of the people while obeying God, ever pressing on to the Promised Land: ". . . for he endured, as seeing Him who is unseen" (Heb. 11:27).

Moses followed God by faith. We emulate his example today. Nothing has changed. Hardships certainly haven't. Wilderness journeys are about the same too. And we know, according to Hebrews 13:8, that Jesus Christ is the same yesterday, today, and forever. If, like Moses, we keep firmly in our mind's eye the one who gave his life for us, we will never fail. We may stumble along the way (when we look away), but we will never fall.

> The only disability in life is a bad attitude.
>
> Scott Hamilton

The Two-Sided Mirror

One of the tools I (Cynthia) use to get in shape is a mirror. The best tonic I can take for indulging in gluttony and laziness is a look in a mirror. I head down to Mervyn's Department Store, grab a swimsuit off the rack (any style will do), put it on, and step in front of the dressing room's three-way mirror. Lord, have mercy! I don't know I've put on that many pounds until I look in that mirror. It helps me see what I really look like. No more "vain imaginings" that I look better than I do. The three-way mirror also shows me my blind spots. I can't see my fanny very well. The mirror helps me see that I need to do a few more bun busters.

I have a love-hate relationship with my mirror, don't you? I hate what it reveals, but I need it to guide me in my dressing—this looks good with that but not with those. Mirrors can be useful tools. If I was out in the forest, I could use one to start a campfire (don't tell Smokey the Bear!) by reflecting the sun in it.

We have a spiritual mirror that does these things and more for us spiritually: the Bible. I can start spiritual fires by reflecting the Son in my life. God's Word tells me everything I know about my Lord. As I focus on him, I become like him. God's Word guides me in dressing my soul. "Clothe yourselves with humility toward one another," 1 Peter 5:5 reads. God's Word reveals *my* blind spots. It's so easy to read Scripture and think it's talking about someone else.

"Oh, that passage reminds me so much of Betty. She definitely has a pride problem!"

God's Word is a mirror that shows me what I am really like. No vain imaginings—God's Word reveals truth. I'm deceived when I believe something else. But the beauty of the Bible is that it's a two-way mirror: on one side reflecting me, but on the other reflecting the loveliness of Jesus Christ.

> But we all, with unveiled face, beholding as in a mirror the glory of the Lord, are being transformed into the same image from glory to glory.
>
> 2 Corinthians 3:18

The longer I gaze into the mirror of God's Word, the more I'll become like Jesus Christ.

Training Togs

We need special shoes and clothes when we begin the walk of faith. Our feet are to be shod "with the preparation of the gospel of peace" (Eph. 6:15). Have you walked anywhere to spread the gospel lately? You really don't have to go far . . . just next door to your neighbor's house. Another use for our spiritual shoes is to run away from sin. What did Joseph (an Old Testament type of Christ) do when Potiphar's seductive wife tempted him to sin? He ran for his life! And that's what the Bible tells us to do each and every time Satan tempts us. Flee immorality (1 Cor. 6:18), flee youthful lusts (2 Tim. 2:22), flee idolatry (1 Cor. 10:14), flee the love of money (1 Tim. 6:10–11). Keep on a-runnin' and don't look back! Do your power walking by fleeing sin and then taking the gospel to the world around you. These two activities will give you a spiritual workout to make you fit for eternity.

Wondering what to wear for spiritual fitness? Clothe yourself with humility (1 Peter 5:5), with Christ (Gal. 3:27), and with the armor of God (Eph. 6:11–17).

I do appreciate the spiritual "girdle" that God has provided. Did you know that we have one? It fits under our clothes, right next to our hearts like a suit of armor, or so the Bible calls it:

> Be strong in the Lord and in the might of His strength. . . . Therefore, take up the full armor of God, so that you will be able to resist in the evil day, and having done everything, to stand firm. Stand firm therefore, *having girded your loins with truth, and having put on the breastplate of righteousness,* and having shod *your feet with the preparation of the gospel of peace;* in addition to all, taking up the shield of faith with which you will be able to extinguish all the flaming arrows of the evil one. And take *the helmet of salvation,* and the sword of the Spirit, which is the word of God.
>
> Ephesians 6:10, 13–17 (emphasis added)

The armor of God strengthens me for the battle I'm engaged in—spiritual combat with a destroyer. We have to know our enemy. First Peter 5:8 calls Satan our adversary, a roaring lion who prowls around seeking someone to devour.

Athletes must always be prepared for the contest and know the obstacles along the way. They overtrain, running more miles in training than are planned for the day of the race. They study the course to be aware of what lies ahead. In similar fashion, we need to be prepared for spiritual warfare with our enemy, Satan. If we are actively serving Christ, the battles and attacks will come. Our spiritual armor will protect and strengthen us for these skirmishes. And in Christ, we will win!

Timely Advice

We need a timepiece to keep us punctual and to gauge our exercise time. Scripture tells us to watch the time spiritually too, redeeming it. "Therefore be careful how you walk, not as unwise men but as wise, making the most of your time, because the days are evil" (Eph. 5:15–16).

Last-days prophecies are being fulfilled at a furious pace during this time in history. The return of Christ is closer by the day. We need to wake up and realize that our appointment with him (for we shall all stand before him) is fast approaching. Are we ready?

> Do this [love one another], knowing the time, that it is already the hour for you to awaken from sleep; for now salvation is nearer to us than when we believed. The night is almost gone, and the day is near. Therefore let us lay aside the deeds of darkness and put on the armor of light.
>
> Romans 13:11–12

Spiritual Weight Lifters

Working out with weights will equip you to carry more of a burden when necessary. As an attractive, feminine lady, you may not want a physical body with big muscles, but it pays to have the strength to do what's needed.

As Christians, we definitely want to build up our spiritual strength too. The Bible offers us weight-lifting advice. There are two types of weight Scripture tells us to carry:

Carry our cross.
Carry others' burdens.

How do we exercise the spiritual strength necessary to lift these burdens? God's Word gives us some clues for lifting each of these weights.

Carrying Our Personal Cross

In Matthew 16:24, Jesus said, "If anyone wishes to come after Me, he must deny himself, and take up his cross and follow Me." Do you have any crosses to bear in your life? Perhaps it's the pain of a difficult marriage. Or the never-ending job of raising a houseful of kids for the Lord. Do you suffer from a chronic illness? Are you the only Christian at your office?

Scripture says not to whine and complain about it, but to bear it. Don't give up, but persevere. Don't give in, but deny yourself instead.

> For whoever wishes to save his life shall lose it; but whoever loses his life for My sake shall find it. . . . For the Son of Man is going to come in the glory of His Father with His angels; and *will then recompense every man according to his deeds.*
>
> Matthew 16:25, 27 (emphasis added)

Jesus denied himself by giving up his glory in heaven and heading toward the cross (Phil. 2:5–8). He did it out of love for us. "Greater love has no one than this," Jesus said, "that one lay down his life for his friends" (John 15:13). Our Lord wants us to prove our love for him by denying ourselves, laying down our lives in service to him through service to others.

Got troubles in your marriage? Feel like throwing in the "His and Hers" towels? Deny your feelings. Hang in there. Be Christ to that spouse, and on judgment day, the Lord will reward you for it.

Struggling to raise kids right? Persevere. Galatians 6:9 encourages us, "Let us not lose heart in doing good, for in due time we will reap *if we do not grow weary*" (emphasis added).

Persecuted at work for your beliefs? "Rejoice and be glad," Jesus said, "for your reward in heaven is great; for in the same way they persecuted the prophets who were before you" (Matt. 5:12).

Bearing Another's Burdens

Carrying our brothers' burdens is the other way that we are commanded to be spiritual weight lifters. When you get too tired to carry your burdens, I need to help you. When I get too tired, you help me. There's no shame in needing assistance on occasion. After all, even Jesus needed help. Yes, he bore the cross for us, but along the way it became too heavy for our Lord. For whatever reason—weakness of body or spirit, heaviness of the load, roughness of the road—he stumbled, and the Roman soldiers recruited Simon of Cyrene to help carry Jesus' cross to Calvary.

When your illness gets you down emotionally as well as physically, I need to minister to you. Bring dinner. Drive you to doctors' appointments. Research your condition on the Internet. Provide a listening ear and a shoulder to cry on. Play with your kids. Anything supportive that will give you hope and lift your spirits. I need to carry your burden until you gain spiritual and physical strength again.

A beautiful example of this concept is found in Exodus 17. Joshua was leading Israel into battle against the Amalekites. Moses, Aaron, and Hur stood on a mountain overlooking the valley as Israel went to war. Moses, the staff of God in one hand, held his arms up over the battling armies. It was like a life-and-death college football game. As long as Moses' hands remained high, the Israelites were ahead; when his arms drooped with fatigue, they fell behind and the Amalekites prevailed. Aaron stuck a rock under the weary leader so Moses could sit down. Then Aaron and Hur came alongside him and held his arms up, one on each side. With their help, Moses' hands stayed steady until the victory was won.

I (Cynthia) recently had a dear friend do this for me. I was going through a very difficult time. Ana lives in another town and was unaware of my problems, but the Holy Spirit spoke to her heart and she telephoned me.

"Cindy, in prayer this morning God revealed that you are going through difficulties," she said. "I'm fasting and praying for you today."

It was such a beautiful deed, and I pray her reward is great. Because of health problems, I couldn't fast at that time. My friend did it for me. Tiny Ana "held up my arms" in prayer and fasting until the victory was won! "Bear one another's burdens, and thereby fulfill the law of Christ" (Gal. 6:2).

When we carry our weights for Christ, we build spiritual muscles that only come from the discipline of obedience. The blessings that result for ourselves and for others far outweigh any momentary burden on us.

9

R and R for Life Balance

Here we are near the end of the book, and again we must return to the beginning: When God created the earth, he worked six days. Then on the seventh day, the almighty Creator rested. In doing so, he established a pattern for us to follow: Work, then rest, work, then rest . . .

It's an example of a balanced life. Balance for each day, each week, each year. Balance for a lifetime. In the beginning of your life, one of your greatest needs was rest. Newborns sleep an average of fourteen to sixteen hours a day. Little ones require this extra slumber due to their rapid growth stage. Besides, they've traveled a long journey to get here!

In the same way, you are traveling a long journey as you follow the Lord and become the best you can be inside and out. One of your greatest needs is rest too. Both body and soul require time to relax and renew. In the next few pages, we'll share some ways to find refreshment for the total you.

Bedtime Blues

"The beginning of health is sleep," an Irish proverb has reminded us for years. We need to take this truth to heart.

Many beneficial functions occur in those precious hours each night when you enjoy suspended consciousness. While you are sleeping, your body and brain are repairing, restoring, rebuilding, and healing themselves. Research has shown that in NREM (dreamless) sleep, while you are motionless in bed, your body is actually very active. During this time, it repairs and regenerates cells, builds bones and muscles, and strengthens the immune system. In sleep, the human growth hormone (HGH) is released, revitalizing your physical and mental health, renewing your energy, and keeping you young.

Insufficient sleep causes many problems, such as daytime fatigue and grogginess, slowed reaction time, lack of mental acuity, irritability and inability to cope, spaciness, and generalized body pain and achiness. Sleep deprivation for longer than three days results in weakness, immune system dysfunction, and even hallucinations and psychoses. In a Great Britain sleep study, weight lifters were allowed only three hours of sleep a night. The plan was to test them for three nights, but after the second night with such little sleep, the athletes couldn't even complete their normal set of presses, lifts, and curls.

When you don't sleep at night, your immune system takes a night off. Dr. Carol Everson, Ph.D., a neurobiology researcher at the University of Chicago, discovered that chronic sleep deprivation caused the immune system to ignore abnormal levels of bacteria in the body, allowing them to proliferate.[1] Insomniacs and others who get minimal sleep demonstrate a reduction in T cells and other disease-fighting cells, according to a study done at the University of California, San Diego.[2] That's why you are more susceptible to illness when you are running around like crazy and beginning to get that "run-down feeling."

Creating Creative Genius

While your body sleeps, your brain is very active. Genuine, healing rest comes in five stages. The first four levels of sleep are named after letters of the Greek alphabet: alpha, beta, theta, delta. These levels take you from drowsiness to deep sleep. In the delta stage, physical restoration transpires. In the fifth and last stage, REM (rapid eye movement) sleep, dreams occur. Studies concur that this is the most important phase of sleep, a necessary time when the brain commits to memory events of the day, creates new ideas, and sorts out problems and solutions for survival. Ever go to bed with a problem and wake up with the answer? For that, you can thank God for creating the REM stage of sleep!

The brain is ready to create when refreshed by REM sleep. Writers and other artists know that the mind is sharpest in the early hours after waking. Novelists and other literary masters have found that they create their best work just after rising in the morning. Another theory also proposes that REM sleep keeps the brain sharp by activating nerve networks, preventing atrophy.

It seems that the reason sleep deprivation can cause hallucinations and psychoses is the brain's need for dreaming. When it is deprived of this natural musing, the brain provides a way to create a dreamlike state. One theory states that REM sleep helps us work on subconscious complications and emotional issues. Keep a dream diary in your "New You" notebook. Jot down the details of the previous night's dream upon waking and analyze the meaning. You may be subconsciously working out a problem in your life.

Cynthia Shares

I had specific dreams growing up. The big ones were that I would have five kids, that I would be a writer and communicator, that I would win others to Christ, and that I would have a healing retreat center and help others get well in body and soul. There were other smaller dreams along the way: the place in the country, the house that looked like a castle that we couldn't afford (but it was in the Father's plan), the family ministry trip around the United States, the trips to Mexico, and so many more.

Spiritually, you also need dreams. God places his purpose in your heart as you are maturing. As you follow him closely, the Lord will begin to develop his plan, allowing events to unfold in your life as only God Almighty can. Look at the life of Joseph. As a boy he had big dreams. He was ridiculed when he shared these dreams with his family. Yet God moved through circumstances to make those prophetic dreams come true.

Use your "New You" notebook to record the dreams of your heart. Write them down in detail and leave room to date God's fulfillment. Remember the saying, "Whatever you can conceive and believe, you can achieve."

> All our dreams can come true—if we have the courage to pursue them.
>
> Walt Disney

Add God to the equation, and the sky is the limit! Remember his promise, "Delight yourself in the LORD; and He will give you the desires of your heart" (Ps. 37:4). In our next LifeBalance book, *The Inner Balance,* we offer our readers specific ways to delight themselves in the Lord. Not only will your relationship with Christ be particularly satisfying, but your entire life will be blessed beyond measure!

Charity Chats

From my earliest years of life, I was known as the little girl with big dreams. At the age of four, I could communicate in colorful detail the dreams God had placed in my heart and the special plan I believed he had for my life. "I'm gonna be a singer and sing songs about Jesus, and I'm gonna talk to people and tell them that Jesus loves them. I'm gonna be on the radio and on TV, and people who don't know Jesus will hear about him 'cause I'll tell them," went my zealous mantra.

Twenty-four years later, the mantra has been refined a bit, but the dream remains exactly the same: to use the gifts of communication that God has given me, in word and in song, to lead the lost to the love of the Savior. This passionate dream has propelled my life since childhood and been a life force that has given me the drive to overcome seemingly overwhelming obstacles and the courage to travel the treacherous, narrow road of a Christian living in Hollywood. The journey has not been easy but has been worth every step thus far as I have seen dreams fulfilled, God glorified, and my character changed. I am young, and many of my dreams have not yet come to fruition, but I have faith that God placed these dreams in my heart for a reason and that his purposes will be fulfilled in his good time.

In recent years, I have become passionate about speaking to young people about the power of believing in their dreams. God has recently taught me a new truth about dreams that I want pass on to you: Dreams *are* powerful, but they are not our own. Dreams belong to the Lord. They are his to give, his to take away, and his to transform. If we understand this and submit our lives to his agenda, nothing can limit what can be done with *his dreams* at work in our lives! So take it from the "Eternal Dreamer" and dream on!

Live Long

It's been proven: Hours in bed add years to your life. So set that alarm for later. Curl up in a quilt and catch a few more moments of shut-eye. A famous study from Alameda County, California, revealed that people who sleep longer live longer. In the study, men who slept seven to eight hours a night and women who slept six to seven hours a night had a much lower mortality risk than those who slept less.[3]

Our bodies were created to respond to the circadian rhythm, the cycle of sunrise and sunset. As darkness descends around us, we produce the hormone melatonin, increasing our desire for sleep. At sunrise, our adrenals release the hormone cortisol to give us energy for our day. Obviously, it's intended that when the sun goes down, we lay down, and went it pops up, so do we. In 1879, however, Thomas Edison invented the lightbulb. Since that time, life has changed, and so have our sleep patterns. The average amount of sleep has gone from nine hours per night to under seven.

In actuality, we should spend one-third of our lives in bed. If it sounds like a waste of time, think again—it may add years to your life. According to William Dement, M.D., Ph.D., director of the Stanford Sleep Disorder Clinic and chairman of the National Commission on Sleep Disorders Research, the single most important determinant in predicting longevity—more influential than diet, exercise, or heredity—is healthy sleep.[4]

Guaranteed Shut-Eye

If fulfilling your body's requirements for sleep has been difficult lately, here are some ideas that may help:

Create comfort. Sleep in a cool, dark, quiet room with good ventilation. If you prefer weight on your bed, invest in a down comforter. Change sheets often; wash with fabric softener. Purchase comfortable, attractive silky pajamas or warm flannel gowns to cuddle up in. Wear cotton socks if your feet get cold at night. Do whatever it takes to make bedtime a temptation!

Unwind. Before bed, watch TV (nothing too stimulating!), glance through a magazine, listen to music, or read a book or your Bible.

Don't indulge. Do without food or beverages three hours before retiring. Going to bed on a full stomach can make you grumble all night. Remember that birthday dinner where you were forced to overeat? After all, you were celebrating, right? But you paid for the celebration all night with stomach pain. Indigestion and gas are just two of the problems late-night binging can produce. We won't mention extra pounds! If you drink before bed, especially caffeinated drinks, you'll be up all night visiting the loo, with inevitable sleep disturbances. Plus, caffeinated drinks are stimulants that may prevent you from falling asleep at all.

Tryptophan. An amino acid that causes drowsiness, tryptophan can be found in turkey, bananas, and milk. If you have trouble falling asleep, try this natural remedy: a low-fat banana milkshake!

Aromatherapy. Health practitioners have used aromatherapy for centuries to bring about healing states. Essential oils evoke a response in the central nervous system and brain. Depending on the fragrance, the reaction can be stimulating or calming. Here are some scents that make sense for sleeping:

> *Cedarwood.* Cedar is mentioned in the Bible and is known for its relaxing, meditative properties.
>
> *Clary Sage.* This old fragrance will unwind your body and comfort your soul.

Eucalyptus. This tree oil promotes sleep.

Frankincense. One of the gifts the Magi brought the Christ child, this incense is recorded in Scripture twenty-one other times. It has calming properties.

Lavender. This scent has a balancing effect on the body and mind.

Patchouli. This essence is a sedative in large amounts and calms and warms the body and soul.

Rose. The scent of this favorite flower will comfort and uplift. It brings to mind happy memories in Grandma's garden.

Herbs and Teas. In Asia, herbal teas have been used for centuries in culturally important, relaxing rituals. An ancient Chinese proverb praises tea in this way: "Better to be deprived of food for three days than of tea for one." The Japanese tea ceremony includes four reflective principles: harmony, respect, purity, and tranquility. Perhaps you would like to establish your own private "tea ceremony" for bedtime or any time of day when you want to relax. Here are some herbs that promote relaxation:

Chamomile. This tea has a calming, sedative effect.

Lemon Verbena. Also boasting a calming influence, this tea came to us from France.

Green Tea. Packed with antiaging antioxidants, this tea has less caffeine than coffee or black tea. But at night, use decaffeinated.

Fruit-Flavored Herbal Teas. Good before bed, these teas have no caffeine. Because they are naturally aromatic with fruit essences, you use less stimulating sugar for flavoring.

Exercise. Adding exercise to your day burns extra energy and promotes sleep at night. Studies have found that exercising in the early evening—for example, taking that stroll after dinner—improves the quantity and quality of your sleep. (Stay away from strenuous exercise just before bed, though. It can keep you awake.) Also recommended is slow-moving yoga to stretch out and relax. The habit of deep breathing will carry over into your sleep time and draw life-giving oxygen into your body.

Massage. Study at the Touch Research Institute at the University of Miami Medical School found a thirty-minute neck massage reduces depression, lowers levels of stress hormones cortisol and norepinephrine, and improves quality of sleep.[5] Just think what a one-hour, whole-body massage will do! Your husband just might agree to a trade. Offer to do him first though, or it's counterproductive!

Sex. Ask your husband if he sleeps better after love making. Okay, maybe he's not an objective person to query. But researchers have found that intimacy at bedtime promotes restful sleep. Of course, the researchers were men too! But try it and see if the "cure" works for you. (Research has proven that satisfying sex between a loving husband and wife, as God intended, promotes good health and longevity. Studies show that married people live longer. Work on that relationship!)

Journaling. Write tomorrow's "To Do" list on a tablet and leave it on the breakfast table. You'll sleep better. No need to worry about things to do and appointments to keep the next day. In addition, the habit of emptying your mind before bed into a journal (or your "New You" notebook) promotes peaceful sleep. Release pent-up emotions onto the empty page and leave them there. Head the page, "Dear Lord" instead of "Dear Diary." You really can trust Jesus Christ with your deepest secrets. He's a faithful, confidential friend who will stay with you for life, and beyond!

Prayer. You can also practice the habit of prayer before sleeping. That way you leave your concerns with him. God's awesome power is at work on the problem while you're sleeping. True rest comes from the Lord.

> When you lie down, you will not be afraid;
> When you lie down, your sleep will be sweet.
>
> Proverbs 3:24

> The fear of the LORD leads to life,
> So that one may sleep satisfied, untouched by evil.
>
> Proverbs 19:23

Meditation. Memorize Scripture as you fall asleep. Meditate on it (mull it over), allowing the Holy Spirit to work on your heart and mind while you are "out."

Daytime Rest Times

After you have established healthful nighttime sleep rituals, begin to find times in the day to take restorative breaks. Hard work is good for the body and soul. America was built on vigorous, responsible labor. We need pauses throughout our workdays to refresh and renew, however, to make us more effective. In the following pages, we offer healthy habits that you may want to establish.

Napping

Alexandra Stoddard, author of *Living a Beautiful Life,* has said that "far too many people, conscientious, ambitious and hard-working, won't, for whatever reason, give themselves permission to have a moment's peace."[6] Isn't this true in the society we live in? If we aren't producing, we aren't important. Jill Murphy Long has written a delightful little book entitled *Permission to Nap.* It's sprinkled with graceful art, soothing sayings, and welcome advice. She encourages Westerners to add napping to their lives. Only in our American world is a daily siesta a cultural crime. Whenever we've traveled south of the border, shopkeepers close up in the middle of the day to take their healthy time-outs. And our disdain of midday dozing has a double standard. Ever notice that it doesn't cross gender lines? Your dad or husband or favorite great-uncle can snooze in a roomful of people, snoring shamelessly, and it rouses nothing but a mere chuckle. Let you or your mom do it, and you're declared lazy and unfit for productive womanhood. I bet Proverbia found her strength and energy in a noontime break. The writer of Proverbs just forgot to include that fact in the record!

Don't feel guilty about getting some rest in the middle of your busy day if you need it. Take ten or fifteen minutes at work (skip the coffee break!) to stretch out on the floor with your pillow (kept in an office cupboard) and benefit from a power nap. At home, curl up with a cotton quilt or woven throw. Lie down by the fireplace and allow the flickering flames to lull you into Dreamland. Even if you have a houseful of noisy kids, insist that they have a quiet time to rest, read, or watch an inspirational movie. When I (Cynthia) was sick, I used to tell my kids, "Don't disturb me during this hour unless you are bleeding!" The quiet-time ritual will bring security to your kids plus restoration to their harried mom. Virginia Woolf once said, "There is a luxury in being quiet in the midst of chaos." Moms, live luxuriously!

Some secrets for successful siestas:

Position is important. Lie down with your feet up.

Get comfortable. You don't want binding clothing or shoes to disrupt your beauty sleep.

Get quiet. Close the door and curtains. Take the phone off the hook. Threaten (or bribe, whichever is your style) the kids or coworkers. Put a "Do Not Disturb" sign on the front door. If noise is a problem in your neighborhood, try a soothing, continuous-play CD (some come with "nature sounds") or even ear plugs.

Eat light. You want a little food on your stomach so hunger doesn't wake you. A carb meal can promote drowsiness. Don't you often feel sleepy after lunch? But feeling stuffed does not promote satisfying sleep either.

Know your nap time. Each person has a certain number of minutes of naptime that work best for their bodies. An hour does my (Cynthia's) body good—and when I was sick, I required it. Now I am so healthy and busy I rarely need a nap. My husband, on the other hand, can't sleep more than ten or fifteen minutes or he wakes up grouchy. At least, that's the excuse he gives! I (Charity) usually aim for fifteen to thirty minutes, the average nap times that benefit most people. It's enough sleep to refresh and reenergize me without disrupting my nightly sleep pattern.

Bed-Free Breaks

Here are some ideas to provide *Healthy Balance* pauses in your day when you're not near a bed:

Listen to classical music or other favorite tunes.

Take a scenic drive up the coast or into a mountain forest. Absorb the natural sounds: waves lapping, seagulls calling. Or savor the rich silence of the woods. Breathe deeply of misty, salt-flavored air or the Christmas scent of pines. Close your eyes and allow the nostalgia to transport you to seasonal childhood memories.

Enjoy a movie with a happy ending—the boy gets the girl, the girl gets well, and good prevails over evil.

Work up a sweat and release some morphine-like endorphins by participating in your favorite sport or aerobic activity.

Hobbies are wonderful distractions from pain, illness, and complex situations.

Escape to a hot bubble bath complete with candles and delightful fragrances.

Schedule a massage. A thorough rubdown gives your circulatory system the equivalency of a five-mile walk. Which would you rather indulge in? Either choice is a wonderful time-out.

Get involved in a lively discussion. Nothing takes your mind off worries like a good debate among friends. And if you're discussing heavenly matters, all the better. You can swap stories of all God is teaching you and grow spiritually in the process.

Laugh Lines

I (Cynthia) actually love my laugh lines. They show a part of my personality that I'm proud of—my sense of humor. In this way, I take after my dad. No matter the situation, he can always joke about something. His quick wit has softened many blows, whether his own on us or life's on him: Yes, he was a firm believer in corporal punishment, but he'd always laugh heartily when delivering his message to us!

No one loves a good laugh more than me. It's in my genetic makeup. And when I discovered the healthy benefits of laughter, I upped my daily quota of belly laughs. My immune system needs all the help it can get. Giggles and guffaws raise your levels of Immunoglobulin A, the immune complex famous for protecting your mucus membranes, your body's first line of defense. Laughter also releases cytokines, which promote vigorous activity of the natural killer cells in your blood. Besides, a good chuckle is like a massage for your insides, stimulating your vital organs and improving blood flow.

Laughter is a body and mind stress buster. It lifts both body and soul, causing you to breathe deeply, and it also relaxes muscles and reduces anxiety, tension, and depression.

> Learn to feel joy.
>
> Seneca
> (4 B.C.–A.D. 65)

Got pain? Laughter increases the release of endorphins, nature's powerful painkillers. Chuckles stimulate the brain centers that tell us to feel good (serotonin, the pleasure hormone, is also released), and they block pain signals in the brain temporarily. Norman Cousins wrote the book *Anatomy of an Illness,* which describes how he healed himself of an agonizing connective tissue disease through daily doses of humor. He rented old comedy videos and snickered his way back to health!

Scripture supports Cousins's findings. Proverbs 17:22 says, "A merry heart does good, like medicine" (NKJV). These ideas just might give you something to smile about:

Comics. I (Cynthia) never read the comics until recently. I felt it was a waste of time. My motto: on to the hard news! But I've changed my opinion now. The Sunday comic section adds levity to my week and gives me a lighthearted perspective on life. I have my favorites—Peanuts, Garfield, Cathy, and B.C. They have never failed to give me a good laugh before I head off to church. Sometimes they remind me of friends or recent situations we've been in. I cut the cartoons out to stick in the mail. I want my friends to receive the healthful benefits of laughter too!

Cartoons. Most cartoons, whether big or small screen, were made with the purpose of evoking laughter. Watch them with your kids. Laugh heartily. Your children will love it! And you'll be nurturing both you and them. One early Saturday morning, my (Cynthia's) youngest son and I laughed so hard at Sylvester the Cat that we woke his dad up with our levity. Looney Tunes are my personal favorite. The jokes are clever enough to satisfy my more sophisticated funnybone, but the slapstick sends the kids (and my husband) into hysterics.

Jokes. A joke a day keeps the doctor (and psychiatrist) away! Wholesome witticisms can give you the encouragement you need. Read or watch humorists like Erma Bombeck, Mark Twain, Bill Cosby, Robin Williams, Barbara Johnson, Liz Curtis Higgs, or Becky Freeman. Buy a joke book or trade puns and banter with friends and coworkers. We have a longtime family friend, Vern Bentz, who keeps our crew supplied with clean jokes. He always brings a new laugh when he visits, and he lifts our spirits in the process.

Amusement. My (Charity's) husband and I plan "play nights." Once a month we visit a clean comedy sports club and laugh until our bellies ache. Nothing compares to laughing together! A favorite family friend and former pastor, David Sotelo, always provides a good laugh with his off-the-cuff humor. And his fun is free!

Find joy in the creation. Watch people, not to criticize, but to recognize human nature in them. Learn to laugh at yourself. That way, you'll never run out of things to amuse you, and you'll beat others to the punch! Look at the other side of a situation to see if there's something humorous in it.

Speaking of other people, soothe awkward or uncomfortable situations with a light heart. Tell a joke. Proverbs 15:1 says, "A soft answer turns away wrath" (NKJV). Levity lightens angry attitudes and tears down walls of pride. It can open doors of communication. Scripture does also say to "speak the truth in love" (Eph. 4:15), but truth is like strong medicine. Taken in small doses, it heals and restores health. However, when an overdose is taken, it's lethal!

Treat others as gently as you want to be treated. Offer them grace, but always stay faithful to the truth. This merits repeating: Follow Jesus' example when he told the woman caught in adultery, "Neither do I condemn you; go and sin no more" (John 8:11 NKJV). His words were few, but they released that woman to live a life of freedom and forgiveness.

You can find something to smile at in all of life. After all, God must have a sense of humor. He created monkeys, giraffes, anteaters—and us!

Our Creator loves our joy, even commands it. We do ourselves a favor and please him too when we discover small things to laugh at daily.

If you are going through a difficult time, do what Scripture requests and offer your joy as "a *sacrifice* of praise" to the Lord (Heb. 13:15, emphasis added). A sacrifice means that it's costly and not easy for you to do. When you count your trials as joy as James 1 commands, it brings great pleasure to your God and King. Your happiness makes your Creator happy.

When I was sick and bedridden, this was true for me (Cynthia). My children's laughter in the other room lifted my spirits. My daughters' sweet, singing voices would bring a smile to my face. And every so often, each of my sons would creep into my room to brighten my day with a funny story or joke. I knew that my contentment in my painful circumstances brought a smile to my Lord's face too. I penned this prayer in my journal:

> Lord, to You I offer my laughter.
> As a gift, I give You my joy.
> It is an act of worship, a sacrifice of praise.
> I certainly don't feel like laughing and praising . . .
> But
> Help me to know that my deep gladness delights
>   You, my Father.
> If I can know joy in the midst of this pain, You are
>   pleased.

Rest for the Soul

You can do all the right things—eat right, sleep tight, exercise regularly, and get to bed early at night. But if you don't have rest for your soul, you'll never be truly healthy. Creator God knew this and established the pattern of the Sabbath. He made it a law, the fourth commandment, so his creation would obey and find renewal for their bodies and souls:

> Remember the sabbath day, to keep it holy.
>
> Exodus 20:8

> For six days work may be done, but on the seventh day there is a sabbath of complete rest, holy to the LORD; whoever does any work on the sabbath day shall surely be put to death.
>
> Exodus 31:15

Who would disobey a law if the punishment was death? That's how important God knows the Sabbath rest is. And yet, even though we Christians realize the value of the Sabbath rest, we don't abide by it. We are happy when stores don't adhere to the "closed Sundays" policy of yesteryear. That way we can head straight to the mall after church! (Many people go to the mall before church and spend the Lord's day there. At those times, the malls could be called "temples of doom." People are worshiping their true god there—materialism. They won't find eternal life in temples of doom.) We're unhappy when our favorite restaurant suddenly closes on Sundays so the proprietors can "spend time with family." We loved to "fellowship" there with our friends after Sunday service!

~~Cynthia Shares~~

When I was on staff of a large church, Sunday became my busiest work day. I had always loved my Sundays before that, spending them quietly enjoying the Lord and my family. I grew to dread them, however.

These days, I don't have a job on the Lord's Day. But after church, we spend our day in a whirlwind of activity, usually catching up on work we've neglected during the week—the yard, the car, the wash, the homework, the writing assignments.

I've read *Little House on the Prairie*. I know how the Sabbath is really supposed to be celebrated. Back then they did all their work, including the food preparation, on Saturday so they could sit around and read Bible storybooks on Sunday (their house was too far from town to attend church). Laura thought the Sabbath ordeal boring, but at my age it does sound restful . . . something about that no noontime meal prep . . .

Chapters 3 and 4 of Hebrews are the "rest chapters" of the Bible. One of the Greek words for rest found in chapter 4 is *sabbatismos*. Spiros Zodhiates' *Complete Word Study Dictionary New Testament* explains that *sabbatismos* is a divine rest, the Sabbath rest that God established in the beginning. We modern-day Americans don't understand Sabbath rest at all. Our weekends are lived at the same breakneck pace as the rest of our week.

Chuck Smith, founder of Calvary Chapels, believes the Sabbath is meant to be spent in bed. Scripture repeatedly calls it "complete rest." But to be complete, something has to encompass body and soul. We can plan physical rest periods into our lives. Many denominations do. The restful soul is another story, isn't it? People from all walks of life—people who have everything money can buy—cannot find rest for their souls. Over and over in the Old Testament, it's plainly stated that God gives rest. Rest from labor. Rest from the journey. Rest from attacking enemies. Rest for people and rest for the land.

God told David, a man of war, that he was giving him a son who would be a man of rest. Solomon's name means "peaceful." The rest that the Lord gives is a peace that passes all understanding. It's this peace of mind and heart that allows us to truly rest at night when we lay our heads on our down pillows. Ecclesiastes 2:23 says about the evil, foolish man who doesn't regard God, "Even at night his mind does not rest." The writer goes on to praise God. Everything good including peace and rest and enjoyment is from his hand. That brings us to the seventh secret of our *Healthy Balance* plan: *Pursue true rest for your body and soul.*

The greatest gift the Father has given us is his own dear Son. Jesus is the answer to our soul's need for rest. In Matthew 11:28–29 he said,

> Come to Me, all who are weary and heavy-laden, and I will give you rest. Take My yoke upon you and learn from Me, for I am gentle and humble in heart; *and you shall find rest for your souls.* (emphasis added)

"Rest" here in the Greek is *anapausis,* which means to give rest, quiet, recreation, and refreshment. The Lord promises us inner tranquility as we go about our daily tasks. The word for "weary" literally means "those who work themselves to exhaustion."

Doesn't this verse sound like it's especially addressed to Americans? Our hectic work schedules aren't all that exhaust us; our recreational pursuits drive us to the brink of craziness too. Have you ever felt more exhausted at the end of your weekend than before it started? How many times have you dreaded going back to work on Monday morning because "I'm just *so* tired?"

Do you saddle yourself with all sorts of expectations, trying to play Superwoman? Do you work night and day to have the spotlessly clean, perfectly decorated home? Are you constantly policing the kids to be sure they mind their manners, dress appropriately, and make you proud? Do you arrive at work early and leave late night after night after night? Are you the church worker whom others can always count on to say yes to commitments? Do you have a heavy burden on your back that you just can't throw off?

Jesus says, "Give it up. Let me take the burden from you. That's not my yoke. My yoke is easy and pleasant. My load is light." A yoke is an agricultural term. Farmers used a yoke to harness two oxen together to plow up ground. The yoke helped them to work side by side in harmony. Jesus is saying, "Yes, I want you to labor with me side by side. We're going to do a great work together. But I'm going to pull most of the weight. I'm stronger than you. Don't try to do more than your share. Besides, my yoke is pleasant and easy. You'll enjoy working with me. And the reason I've yoked myself to you is that I enjoy you. I love you."

The Westminster Confession states, "The chief end of man is to glorify God and enjoy Him forever." When you go to bed at night, you can know peace and true rest. Lie there and fellowship with the Lord. Meditate on how much your Savior loves and enjoys you and praise him for it. Then your greatest accomplishment of the day will be done—time spent with Jesus Christ just cherishing, worshiping, and enjoying him is what he desires most from you.

Genuine rest will come when we enter into God's Sabbath. This divine rest is the Sabbath God himself entered on completion of his creation work. I (Cynthia) understood this well as I finished up this book. Due to the timing of contract signings and writing two books, I, as primary writer, had only one month to write a heavily researched book and get it to our publisher. It was hard, focused, creative work. The whole month I looked forward to November 1, the day after I was to Fed-Ex the manuscript to Revell. That day, I planned to enter into my "Sabbath." I had all sorts of recreational activities planned that day with my youngest son who is still homeschooled. Later that night, I planned to share a celebration dinner with the rest of my family. The day after I finished the manuscript, I got my rest, all right. I caught a bad case of the flu and spent the entire next week in bed. I couldn't have gotten up if I had wanted to! I guess it was God's enforced Sabbath for me. So stay balanced—if you don't, he'll balance you out one way or the other!

The divine rest that God gives us is the same rest that he enjoys. According to Zodhiates, it is ours now as a "present possession and a future blessing." Revelation 14:13 speaks of this promised rest that believers will enter in heaven after being rewarded for earthly deeds done in Christ's name: "They may rest from their labors, for their deeds follow them."

You'll never experience true rest unless you know Jesus Christ personally. The Book of Hebrews, chapter 4, talks about entering into his Sabbath. The work of salvation is accomplished. Jesus Christ paid the price of sin on the cross. "It is finished!" he cried out when atonement was complete. And he bowed his head and died in our place. We no longer have to work for our salvation. It's done. Imagine what it's like for those whose religions teach that a follower must work

Healthy Balance secret #7: Pursue true rest for your body and soul.

and work and work for their own salvation. Their desperate exercise in futility never ends. True rest comes when we trust in Christ and Christ alone for forgiveness of our sins, our relationship with our Creator, and our assurance of eternal life. If we can trust Jesus with our eternity, how much more can we trust him for the everyday problems that keep us awake at night?

As we grow in God's Word and in our relationship with Jesus Christ, it's this trust in his wisdom, strength, and sovereignty that will bring us deep tranquility and genuine rest. The beautifully balanced, strong, and healthy woman is one who radiates the peace of God.

10

The *Healthy Balance* for Life

As you pursue health and fitness, make glorifying God your goal. First Corinthians 6:20 says, "For you have been bought with a price: therefore glorify God in your body."

Charity and I offer our own fitness and nutrition regimens with caution. We don't want any of our readers saying, "This is how Charity and Cynthia get healthy, fit, godly, or beautiful. I'm sure their plan is best for me too." Always talk to your doctor about any specific concerns you have. He or she knows your body and your individual needs. We especially don't want to be put on pedestals or be looked up to as authorities. We are learning along with everyone else. Our bodies are changing and maturing. What works for us today may not work tomorrow. Then we'll have to write another book on the subject!

We always strive for a balance in the areas of fitness and nutrition. It takes supermodels and superstars hours a day and untold amounts of money to produce the figures that wow the world. We couldn't care less about that. Instead, we want to spend as little time and money as possible to maintain all that God has given us, so that we can be the best possible stewards of all his good gifts to us.

We encourage you to find a balance in these areas too. Don't focus only on the kinds of food in your diet, but also think about whether you eat too much or too little. We have given food permission to become an idol in our society, even in the church. Gluttony is an overlooked sin. We turn up our noses at the uncontrolled drunk lying at the doorstep, but the sanctuary is filled with uncontrolled eaters. Scriptures admonish us to use moderation in all things; this includes even the normal, everyday pleasures of good food. It's so easy for our flesh and its appetites to get out of control. But many of us also become obsessed with undereating. We need to maintain a balance in every area, including nutrition.

Believe it or not, we can even become preoccupied with exercise. Anything can take over our lives. Exercise sensibly. It's been said that the flesh is a good servant but a bad master. The apostle Paul knew this. In 1 Corinthians 9:25–27 he says,

> Everyone who competes in the games [Olympics] exercises self-control in all things. They then do it to receive a perishable wreath, but we an imperishable. Therefore I run in such a way, as not without aim; I box in such a way, as not beating the air; but I discipline my body and make it my slave, so that, after I have preached to others, I myself will not be disqualified.

Paul understood that our bodies and appetites could master us and bring us to shame if we allowed them to. He disciplined himself under the power of the Holy Spirit so that he could run the race of life in such a way as to win. We should do the same as we attempt to please the Lord with our lives. Then the weight issue no longer controls us. We can live with our focus on Christ and not on ourselves and our desires. First Corinthians 10:31 is a good motto for our journey:

> Whether, then, you eat or drink or *whatever you do,* do all to the glory of God. (emphasis added)

The Seven Secrets

The seven secrets of the *Healthy Balance* plan will help our stewardship in several areas of our lives: the care of our bodies and minds, our relationships with others, and our souls. Add these rules to your "New You" notebook and review them every day.

1. Learn to love live foods.
2. Practice moderation in all things.
3. Care for others like you care for yourself.
4. Supplement daily with probiotics.
5. Add hope to your life.
6. Learn to love your body in motion.
7. Pursue true rest for your body and soul.

Balanced Living

In America, we make sure our bodies are well fed. In fact, for most of us, well fed becomes too fed! We need to become just as concerned about the condition of our souls. Here is where the *Healthy Balance* comes in. We need to have our lives balanced, taking in spiritual truth as often as we feast on nourishing foods. A religious leader in American history made it his practice to read a passage of Scripture with each meal.

Every time he took in physical sustenance, he also indulged in "spiritual meat." "No time for the Bible, no time for food" was his firm rule. Most of us would be much leaner physically if we followed his example!

Nourishing our spirits makes us strong Christians—guaranteed! We can then exercise our faith through witnessing and serving, and we can enjoy genuine rest for our souls through prayer.

Sustenance for the Journey

"It is good to have an end to journey towards," wrote science fiction author Ursula Le Guin, "but it is the journey that matters in the end."[1] Now as we come to the last pages of our book, you can begin your journey toward wholeness. It may seem like a daunting task, we know. Keep your goals before you, but don't let the prospect of attaining them overwhelm you. The journey is to be appreciated and enjoyed!

If your goal in using the *Healthy Balance* plan is to slim down and get in shape, enjoy the journey. It's fascinating to watch your body transform from soft mush into trim, firm muscles. It's actually fun to chart your weight loss and watch those pounds melt off. (Trust us, it's much more fun than overeating and watching the reverse happen!)

For you who are well but want to take your health and fitness to a new level, we know you can do it. The *Healthy Balance* program provides the nutrients and probiotics, the exercise and renewal habits to ensure your success. All you need to bring to the plan is your commitment, determination, and some perseverance.

For those of you who are ill, the journey toward wellness will take a little longer. A struggle may be ahead for you.

From experience, I (Cynthia) know that you sometimes advance three steps only to fall back two.

Keep in mind that the struggle of climbing the sides of the mountain is developing your inner strength. A perfect picture of this is a butterfly; it needs the struggle of emerging from the pupal stage to build strength in its wings. One time, as an author watched a butterfly labor to free herself from her cocoon, he decided to help the insect. He easily pulled the cocoon away from the butterfly and stepped back to watch. Fully expecting flight, the author was amazed to watch the insect fall to the floor and crawl away. He placed the butterfly in a jar, observing her over several days. The insect never did gain the strength in her wings to fly away, the very thing she was created to do. Through helping, the man had eliminated her struggle, the necessary element to build wings strong enough to fly.

> To live for some future goal is shallow. It's the sides of the mountain that sustain life, not the top.
>
> Robert M. Pirsig

Have you been trapped in a cocoon of extra fat or confining illness? Are you ready to find your freedom? Does it excite you to think of flying away to the heights for which God created you? The strength comes in the struggle. When you stick with the *Healthy Balance* program, persevering no matter what, you will be equipped with everything you need to accomplish all that God has planned for you once you are healthy and fit.

> Happiness is not a state to arrive at, but a manner of traveling.
>
> Margaret Lee Runbeck

Remember to include the Great Physician in your recovery program. My (Cynthia's) health didn't improve until I recognized my dependence on God. He alone could heal me. I asked the Lord to show me how to get well. Second Chronicles tells a story about a king who should have remembered this. Asa was king over Judah. He did good and followed God most of his life. At the end of his life, however, Asa became diseased in his feet. His disease was severe, Scripture tells us. We have to sympathize a little with poor Asa. Life-threatening illness is scary. It's important to get good medical advice, and Asa did . . . he sought doctors and the latest medical treatments. The king didn't commit his condition to God, though. Second Chronicles 16:12–13 records that "even in his disease he did not seek the LORD, but the physicians. So Asa slept with his fathers . . ."

As a follower of Christ, your life is in his hands. In Jeremiah 29:11–14, God says he has plans for your life:

> For I know the plans that I have for you . . . plans for welfare and not for calamity to give you a future and a hope. Then you will call upon Me and come and pray to Me, and I will listen to you. You will seek Me and find Me when you search for Me with all your heart. And I will be found by you . . .

Seek Christ. Ask how he wants you to pursue physical and spiritual health. If his answer includes *The Healthy Balance,* we want to be there to support you and to hear your story. Please stay in touch through mail or e-mail. Commit your way to him and you will always have something inspirational to report!

Whether your goal is fitness, weight loss, or healing, exciting days are ahead. As you work toward your objective, you develop mental and spiritual muscles in addition to training your body. In the near future, you will look back over the miles that you have covered and be truly amazed at what your team of two—God and you—can accomplish. But you must be willing to take that first step. Don't worry about the rest; they will follow. Madame Du Deffand (1696–1780), the marquise influential in the French Revolution, encouraged, "Ah, but in such matters, it is only the first step that is difficult."

Begin the journey toward a healthier you in body and soul, and travel it at your personal pace. As we believers follow the *Healthy Balance* path of nutrition and exercise for body and soul, we'll have the strength and energy to carry out the call of God in our lives. When Christian women are healthy, balanced, and beautiful—serving others for Christ's sake—life on earth will be rich. More importantly, those we've influenced for the kingdom will fill heaven's courts for eternity.

We leave this blessing with you from 1 Thessalonians 5:23:

> Now may the God of peace Himself sanctify you entirely; and may your spirit and soul and body be preserved complete, without blame at the coming of our Lord Jesus Christ.

Notes

Chapter 1: Health

1. Weston A. Price, D.D.S., *Nutrition and Physical Degeneration* (New Caanan, Conn.: Keats Publishing, 1997), 9.

Chapter 2: My Personal Journey to Wellness

1. Dr. C. Orian Truss, "The Missing Diagnosis," *Omni*, March 1985, 44.

Chapter 3: Healthy Balance Foods for Body and Soul

1. David Heber, M.D., *What Color Is Your Diet?* (New York: Regan Books, 2001), xiii.
2. Ibid., 4.

Chapter 4: Lean for Life

1. Roy L. Walford, M.D., *The 120 Year Diet* (New York: Four Walls Eight Windows, 2000).
2. J. Mason, "Nurses' Health Study," *New England Journal of Medicine* 333 (1995): 677.
3. Walford, *120 Year Diet,* 101.
4. *Journal of Nutrition* 133 (January 2003): 1.
5. Charles Stanley, "Soul Food," *In Touch* (March 2003), 40.

Chapter 5: Recipes for a Healthy Balance

1. Study by Barbara Rolls, Ph.D., *Prevention—Women's Health Today* (Emmaus, Pa.: Rodale, 2001), 53.

2. Ibid., 47.

Chapter 6: "I Told You I Was Sick!"

1. Elson Haas, M.D., *The Detox Diet* (Berkeley, Calif.: Celestial Arts, 1996), 7.

2. J. E. Williams, O.M.D., *Viral Immunity* (Charlottesville, Va.: Hampton Roads Publishing, 2002), 112.

3. Michael F. Roizen, M.D., *Real Age* (New York: HarperCollins, 1999), 112.

4. Barry Sears, Ph.D., *Enter the Zone* (New York: Regan Books, 1995), 3.

5. Dr. Jorge Flechas, "Yeast and the CFIDS Patient," *CFIDS Chronicle* (Summer/Fall 1989): 40–42.

6. Dr. Pamela Morford, "The Newest Mystery Illness," *Redbook,* April 1986, 46.

7. W. D. Brodie, *Cancer and Common Sense: Combining Science and Nature to Control Cancer* (White Bear Lake, Minn.: Winning Publications, 1997), 46.

8. Michael Culbert, *Medical Armageddon* (San Diego: C & C Communications, 1995), 69.

9. Roy Walford, *Beyond the 120 Year Diet* (New York: Four Walls Eight Windows), 117.

10. Quoted in Roizen, *Real Age,* 179.

11. C. H. Barrows, Jr., and G. C. Kokkonen, "Dietary Restriction and Life Extension Biological Mechanism," *Nutritional Approach to Aging Research* (Boca Raton, Fla.: CRC Press, 1982), 219.

12. Quoted in Dharma Khalsa, *Food as Medicine* (New York: Simon and Schuster, 2003), 26.

13. Ibid., 3.

Chapter 8: Geared Up for Fitness

1. Spoken message by Dr. Charles Stanley, InTouch Ministries, 1999.

Chapter 9: R and R for a Life Balance

1. Peter Hauri and Shirley Linde, *No More Sleepless Nights* (New York: John Wiley and Sons, 1996).

2. Jill Murphy Long, *Permission to Nap* (Naperville, Ill.: Sourcebooks, 2002), 18–19.

3. Roizen, *Real Age,* 19.

4. Long, *Permission to Nap,* 19.

5. Rolls, *Prevention—Women's Health Today,* 53.

6. Alexandra Stoddard, *Living a Beautiful Life* (New York: Random House, 1996), 39.

Chapter 10: The *Healthy Balance* for Life

1. Ursula LeGuin, *The Left Hand of Darkness* (New York: Ace Books, 2000), 220.

Resources

For Bible Teaching

Precept Ministries International, inductive Bible studies by Kay Arthur
1-800-763-8280 or www.precept.org

InTouch Ministries, teaching by Pastor Charles Stanley
1-800-789-1473 or www.intouch.org

Focus on the Family, teaching by Dr. James Dobson
1-800-661-9800 or www.fotf.org

Thru the Bible Ministries, teaching by Dr. J. Vernon McGee
1-800-65-BIBLE (24253) or www.ttb.org

John Hagee Ministries, resources for faith and healing (including Scripture healing tapes)
1-800-854-9899 or www.jhm.org

For Scripture Memorization

Jack Van Impe Ministries, www. jvim.org

For Further Reading

The Yeast Connection and the Woman by William Crook, M.D. (Professional Books, 1995)

The Gerson Therapy (for cancer) by Charlotte Gerson and Morton Walker, D.P.M. (Kensington Publishing, 2001)

The Power of a Praying Woman by Stormie Omartian (Harvest House, 2003)

The Pursuit of God by A. W. Tozer (Christian Publications, 1993)

Loving God by Charles Colson (Zondervan, 1997)

A Cancer Battle Plan by Anne Frahm (her personal story) (JP Archer, January 1998)

Recovery From Cancer by Eliane Nussbaum (Avery, Penguin Putnam, May 1992)

Books by Dr. Sherry Rogers on nutritional healing, write for list:
Northeast Center for Environmental Medicine
Box 2719
Syracuse, NY 13220-2716
(315) 488-2856 or 467-4458

MIRACLE
MAKEOVERS...

They can happen to you!

Continue your journey
with the latest advice for
body and soul.
Visit our website at

www.lifebalanceladies.com

where you can interact with the authors
in a question-and-answer forum,
preview new releases and LifeBalance products,
and
keep up with the LifeBalance conference
and events schedule.

We hope you'll visit us soon!

The LifeBalance Ladies,

Cynthia   Charity

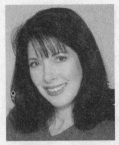

As a researcher for several international health companies, **Cynthia Culp Allen** has a passion to help people of all ages get healthy in both body and soul. She is the award-winning writer of eight hundred articles in newspapers and magazines, including *Mother Earth News*, *Body and Soul*, *Healing Lifestyles and Spas*, *Veggie Life*, *Focus on the Family*, *Brio*, *Guideposts*, *Decision*, and many more. Honored with six national writing awards, Cynthia has written three books: *The Beautiful Balance for Body and Soul* (Revell, 2003) and *The Healthy Balance* (Revell, 2004), both coauthored with her daughter Charity Allen Winters, and *Home Is Where You Hang Your Heart* (Cumberland House, 2002). She has also contributed to eight bestsellers, including *Chicken Soup for the Christian Family Soul* (Health Communications), *The Hidden Hand of God* (Guideposts), *God's Vitamin C for the Hurting Spirit* (Starburst Publishers), *Raising Them Right* (Focus on the Family), and *The NIV Women's Devotional Bible 2* (Zondervan).

Cynthia is a popular speaker for business events, conferences, churches, and retreats, speaking on subjects as diverse as health and nutrition, agriculture, women's topics, parenting, homeschooling, and Christian living. A frequent guest on radio and television, this mother of five lives in northern California with her husband, Charles, and their youngest son, Christian. She stays busy with writing and speaking, homeschooling, running her business (www.culpdiversified properties.com), and taking long walks in the country.

Cynthia can be reached for speaking engagements and guest appearances at (530) 529-4406 or by email at cynthia culpallen@yahoo.com. For more information, please visit www.cynthiaculpallen.com.

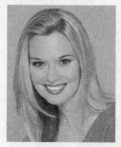

Charity Allen Winters is an established model in the fashion industry. Her print work can be found in such publications as *Allure* magazine, *Sunset*, *Focus on the Family*, *Living with Teenagers*, *Brio*, *Bongos*, and *Model USA*. The rising actress is recognized in Europe as the lead host of *LIFE Television* and has also been featured on many national television shows, including *Just Shoot Me*, MTV, and *Jimmy Kimmel Live*.

As a recording artist with two complete albums, Charity has soloed with the Los Angeles Opera Company and in a variety of television appearances, has opened for country star Charlie Daniels, and was an honored guest in the United Kingdom at a special performance at the Canterbury Cathedral. She is a 1999 graduate of Biola University with a B.A. in mass media communications and a minor in biblical studies.

Charity has spent recent years traveling the country as a national speaker and gospel singer, but she loves coming home to her husband, Kelvin, and serving on her church worship team at the Vineyard Christian Fellowship in Los Angeles. She can be contacted directly for speaking, singing, and guest appearances by email at message4charity@ yahoo.com, or booked through her manager, Paul Webb, at Hollywood Pacific Studios, (818) 349-2093.